The
Vulvodynia
SURVIVAL GUIDE

How to Overcome
Painful Vaginal
Symptoms
& Enjoy an
Active Lifestyle

Howard I. Glazer, Ph.D.
Gae Rodke, M.D., FACOG

NEW HARBINGER PUBLICATIONS, INC.

Publisher's Note

This publication is designed to provide accurate and authoritative information in regard to the subject matter covered. It is sold with the understanding that the publisher is not engaged in rendering psychological, financial, legal, or other professional services. If expert assistance or counseling is needed, the services of a competent professional should be sought.

Care has been taken to confirm the accuracy of the information presented and to describe generally accepted practices. However, the authors, editors, and publisher are not responsible for errors or omissions or for any consequences from application of the information in this book and make no warranty, express or implied, with respect to the contents of the publication.

The authors, editors, and publisher have exerted every effort to ensure that any drug selection and dosage set forth in this text are in accordance with current recommendations and practice at the time of publication. However, in view of ongoing research, changes in government regulations, and the constant flow of information relating to drug therapy and drug reactions, the reader is urged to check the package insert for each drug for any change in indications and dosage and for added warnings and precautions. This is particularly important when the recommended agent is a new or infrequently employed drug.

Some drugs and medical devices presented in this publication may have Food and Drug Administration (FDA) clearance for limited use in restricted research settings. It is the responsibility of the health care provider to ascertain the FDA status of each drug or device planned for use in their clinical practice.

Vulvodynia is a diagnosis that must be made after a careful evaluation by a competent physician. The results cited for diagnostic accuracy and treatment success are based on carefully diagnosed vulvodynia patients who receive personally attended surface electromyographic evaluation and instruction, and close follow-up care to enhance compliance and treat any intercurrent infection or underlying medical condition (such as vaginitis, lichen sclerosus, etc.).

We do not yet have data to support "home evaluation" or treatment by mail order. The devices used require a prescription from a medical doctor, which is a statement of medical appropriateness and necessity.

Distributed in Canada by Raincoast Books.

Copyright © 2002 by Howard I. Glazer and Gae Rodke
New Harbinger Publications, Inc.
5674 Shattuck Avenue
Oakland, CA 94609

Cover design by Poulson/Gluck Design
Edited by Brady Kahn
Text design by Michele Waters

ISBN 1-57224-291-4 Paperback

All Rights Reserved

Printed in the United States of America

New Harbinger Publications' Web site address: www.newharbinger.com

06   05   04

10   9   8   7   6   5   4   3

To my wife, Doreen, and my children, Leslie, Harley, and Ashley. Their patience, love, and enthusiastic support of my work has made this book possible.

—H. Glazer, Ph.D.

To the National Vulvodynia Association in hopes that this book will provide information, comfort, and paths to healing while we continue to work to find causes and cures for this debilitating condition.

—G. Rodke, M.D.

Contents

Acknowledgments

I would like to acknowledge the many people who have taught me, mentored my professional development, supported my work, and aided in the writing of this book.

I would like to thank my mentors: Dr. Abram Amsel, my undergraduate professor at the University of Toronto and my doctoral professor at the University of Texas at Austin, who taught me the rigors of laboratory research and a healthy respect for scientific methodology; Dr. Neal Miller, my post-doctoral professor at the Rockefeller University and the founder of modern day biofeedback; Dr. Herbert Fensterheim, my one and only clinical professor and good friend, who taught me what caring for patients is all about; Dr. John Perry, who introduced me to pelvic floor muscle surface electromyography; and the late Dr. Alexander Young, a founding father in the field of vulvodynia and for many years the director of the Cutaneous Vulvar Center at Columbia University's Department of Dermatology, who introduced me to vulvodynia.

Thanks to the International Society for the Study of Vulvovaginal Disease for welcoming my membership, particularly Dr. Stanley Marinoff, Dr. Libby Edwards, Dr. Jacob Bornstein, Dr. Lynette Margesson, Dr. Harold Michlewitz, and Raymond Kaufman, whose open minds immediately embraced the introduction of an innovative and controversial technology into the treatment of vulvar pain disorders.

Thanks to my institution, the Joan and Sanford Weill Medical College of Cornell University, the New York Presbyterian Hospital, and the departments of psychiatry and of obstetrics and gynecology for their continued support of my work.

Thanks to the National Vulvodynia Association and particularly to its current executive director, Phyllis Mate, and to Christin Veasley, the director of research and development. They have worked long, hard, and selflessly in the pursuit of recognition and support for sufferers of vulvar pain. I am proud to serve as a member of their medical board and continue to support their good works in all possible ways. This book would not have been possible without their efforts.

New Harbinger Publications deserves much credit for their commitment to publishing the first book written specifically for vulvodynia patients. Thanks to Jueli Gastwirth and Brady Kahn, for their enthusiastic support, commitment to this project, and ceaseless efforts to keep things on track throughout the production of the manuscript.

I am most grateful to Kristen Kemp, for her writing efforts and transforming my often unreadable work into what you see in this book.

I thank the Biofeedback Foundation of Europe (www.bfe.org) for their gracious and generous support of my work, including this book.

Finally, I wish to thank all the vulvar pain sufferers who have led me to a better understanding of vulvodynia by sharing their lives and stories with me, both as patients and visitors to my Web site, vulvodynia.com. This book is for all of you.

—H. Glazer

I would like to acknowledge those who have inspired, taught, encouraged, mentored, and supported me in my journey as a student and physician.

Thanks to the University of Arizona College of Medicine and the Albert Einstein College of Medicine of Yeshiva University for their emphasis on teaching the importance of developing clinical skills in medicine; being able to listen and hear the needs of my patients has led me to this area of ongoing study. Two very special professors at the University of Arizona deserve special mention: Dr. Andrew Weil, who gave legitimacy to the field of integrative medicine at a formative period of my learning, and Dr. Peter Lynch, who gave me the vocabulary of dermatology with which to explore the nether regions of gynecology.

Thanks to Dr. Martin Stone, the chairman of my residency program at the University Hospital of the State University of New York at Stony Brook, who recognized my love for ob/gyn and encouraged me to find an area of special interest and continued learning. To my mentor, the late Dr. Eduard Friedrich, for creating the first "Friedrich Fellow in Vulvar Disease," and insisting on doing a "real project" with his new recruit. A special thanks to Dr. Ed Wilkinson for reviewing all those pathology slides gathered through the years, and for his continued friendship and consultation. Both of them supported my nomination and acceptance to the Fellowship of the International Society for the Study of Vulvar Disease (ISSVD), an organization committed to continued sharing and learning of collective wisdom and scientific study. Ongoing thanks to my fellow members, teachers, and mentors in the society, especially Dr. Marilynne McKay, who taught me the importance of "treating conditions" even when a cure was not immediately to be found. Drs. Lynn Margesson, Libby Edwards, and Peter Lynch continue to teach me the best of vulvar dermatology, and I am deeply grateful. To Dr. Benson Horowitz, who has a special knack with unusual "yeast," and Dr. Stanley Marinoff, an excellent surgeon, mentor, and friend. They made it okay to be a practicing gynecologist interested in this area. To Dr. David Foster, who has me more interested in basic scientific research than ever before. And to Dr. Maria Turner for organizing the National Institute of Health conference on vulvodynia and engaging so many scientists from so many disciplines in the collaborative effort to find answers.

Thanks to Dr. Burton Krumholz for allowing me to add vulvar patients to the Colposcopy Clinic roster at Long Island Jewish Medical Center and for teaching me to respect the power of the laser. To Drs. Harold Tovell and Alexander Young, the founders of the Cutaneous Vulvar Service at St. Luke's/Roosevelt Hospital Center for taking me on a seven-year adventure in learning.

Thanks to Marilyn Freedman, physical therapist, who worked with my patients "with all modalities" of physical therapy and gave me the first "positive feedback" on the use of biofeedback for pelvic floor spasm and vulvar pain.

Thanks to Howard Glazer for taking referrals for "pelvic floor rehabilitation with biofeedback" and developing a standardized protocol so that we could systematically treat patients, measure results, and publish data to show that it works.

Thanks to my office staff: to Judy Fuchs, our office manager, for keeping us on track if not always on time; to Helen Rodney and Annette Cleghorn on the front lines and in the back rooms, often simultaneously; and to Abbe Niborski-Nadel and Donna Gunther, our nurse practitioners, who are my right and left hands and extra eyes and ears—and who do it all with great care.

And a very special thanks to my patients who got me started by having problems and conditions for which there were no easy fixes and few resources for referral. Your patience and devotion and ongoing optimism and willingness to share your most intimate triumphs and heartaches with me have kept me trying to help you find answers and relief. Thanks to RB for helping me write the first self-help pamphlet on vulvodynia for the ICA, to DL for starting the New York Metropolitan Vulvodynia Support Group, and to Phyllis Mate and the National Vulvodynia Association for taking the crusade to a national level.

Thanks to Kristen Kemp for harnessing our energies, resources, and jargon, and for helping us speak clearly to the needs of our readers. Many thanks to our editors, Jueli Gastwirth and Brady Kahn, and publisher, New Harbinger Publications, for making it happen.

Last, but by no means least, I wish to thank my husband, best friend, and colleague Dr. Charles Swencionis for his ongoing support, understanding, and contribution to our efforts, especially in the areas of psychophysiology, behavior, and statistics. You are the best.

—G. Rodke

On behalf of the National Vulvodynia Association (NVA), I would like to express my appreciation to Drs. Howard Glazer and Gae Rodke for their commitment to treating vulvodynia patients and for recognizing the need for this book. My heartfelt thanks to the following special people, all of whom I am fortunate to know as friends: Mona Schlossberg, the driving force behind the NVA's creation; Harriet O'Connor, NVA cofounder and volunteer director of support services; Christin Veasley, our indispensable director of research and professional programs; and Maurice Kreindler, the NVA's treasurer and most ardent advocate. I am also grateful to our Executive and Medical Advisory Board members (past and present) and the generous donors who support our work.

—P. Mate
President of the
National Vulvodynia
Association

Introduction

Thousands of women suffer with vulvodynia. To receive maximum relief from this complex syndrome, an integrative approach is necessary. From self-help measures to medication to biofeedback and even surgery, there are many options to help women deal with their pain. We decided to write this book because we want you to know that help is out there. We know that many women are suffering needlessly from vulvovaginal pain. In this book, we outline what you can do to alleviate the pain and get your life back on track.

You are not alone. The two stories that follow—as with all the accounts in this book—are from real women, many of whom we've met through the course of our work. Other stories are from women who've contacted the National Vulvodynia Association. For more stories like these, you can also visit Dr. Glazer's Web site at www.vulvodynia.com.

Jordanna's Ordeal

During her first two years of college, Jordanna had a steady boyfriend with whom she enjoyed making love. She had a healthy attitude toward sex and even considered studying to become a sex therapist. Just before Jordanna's junior year, her doctors found a cyst on her ovary and she underwent successful laparoscopic surgery. Unfortunately, a routine dose of preoperative antibiotics set off a series of yeast infections. Jordanna wasn't too concerned because she was still experiencing a normal sex life and figured the problem would just go away.

At twenty-one, Jordanna became involved with a new boyfriend. She fell in love and was having the best sexual relationship of her life. Then the pain started. It began subtly, with discomfort around the vaginal opening upon penetration. The pain went away when her boyfriend started thrusting, so she assumed she needed more lubrication and applied it each time she made love. To her dismay, lubrication didn't help. Sex started hurting more, rather than less. At the same time, recurring yeast and urinary infections made her problem worse.

After a while, Jordanna began to worry that the pain was all in her head or that she was just too tense. The school's gynecologist seconded that notion by telling her he couldn't find anything wrong. "He told me to have a drink and relax, and things would get better," Jordanna later recalled. He also recommended using more lubrication, but she knew that wasn't the answer.

After graduation, she saw another gynecologist who tried to find the triggers of her vulvar pain. He also said it was probably a lubrication problem and suggested she try different sexual positions that wouldn't put as much pressure on the tissue surrounding the vaginal opening.

For the next two years Jordanna suffered. Sometimes the pain eased up, but other times her vulva hurt so badly that intercourse was impossible. Over time, sex became the last thing she wanted to do and she didn't even want to try nonpenetrative activity. Her libido was waning because sex produced pain.

"I tensed up every time my boyfriend mentioned it," she said. "I knew he wanted to have intercourse, and I felt ashamed, pitiful, depressed, and angry that I couldn't." If she said no, he'd be terribly disappointed; if she agreed, she'd be in terrible pain. She was upset with her body for not cooperating and angry with her boyfriend for pressuring her.

Meanwhile, her vulva began hurting so badly that she was determined to find out what was wrong. "I don't know why it took me so long to find some real answers," she said. She got out a hand mirror and checked out her genitals. "My vulva seemed red and swollen, especially around my opening," she said. Jordanna went to another physician, showing her what she'd found. She even used the doctor's finger to try to show her where the pain was located. Jordanna said the doctor seemed embarrassed by her frankness and told her there was nothing wrong. "It really could be in your head," the doctor said. But the doctor did add, "Or you might have something called vulvodynia." Finally, the doctor referred Jordanna to a physician who specializes in comprehensive vulvar pain evaluations.

Jordanna learned a great deal about her problem, and after extensive testing, she began to get the treatment she needed. Finally, Jordanna had names for her problem: *vulvodynia*, particularly, *vulvar vestibulitis* (VVS), or pain in the vestibule. She repeated them over and over again in her mind when she left the office. She was overwhelmed with relief to learn that her pain was real—not imaginary—it was a recognized syndrome, and treatments were available. She also learned that she was not alone—other women had the same problem, and many of them had seen great improvement following treatment.

Jordanna discovered that up to 15 percent of women have vulvodynia (Goetsch 1991). The disorder is characterized by itching, burning, and painful intercourse. Some women, like Jordanna, only have pain on penetration. Others with VVS experience pain in the vestibule that's easily provoked by tight clothing or sitting. Still more females suffer from other kinds of vulvar pain.

After all of this time, Jordanna had an explanation for herself and her boyfriend. She finally had hope for getting better.

Katherine's Story

Katherine was forty-two years old when she was diagnosed with another kind of vulvodynia: *dysesthetic vulvodynia* (also known as *essential vulvodynia* or *generalized vulvar dysesthesia*). For a few years, she experienced tingling, stinging, and itching in the entire vulvar region, including her labial tissue, clitoris, urethra, perineum, and occasionally on her inner thighs. For her, the pain wasn't constant, but she did experience it on a daily basis. It started out faintly, but the discomfort gradually became more frequent and lasted for longer periods of time. Randomly, she would get temporary relief, but not often. It was always a part of her day and her awareness. Three years ago, she decided to find out what the problem was once and for all. Katherine went to two different doctors, an internist and a gynecologist, and was treated repeatedly for yeast infections. When the problem didn't go away, they sent her to a nearby clinic to be tested for every infection possible—all the tests came back negative.

"After considerable Internet research, I found out about vulvodynia," she said. "But it was terribly embarrassing explaining it to doctors who'd never even heard the term before. They looked at me like I was nuts and told me the problem was in my head." Finally Katherine found a doctor who specialized in vulvodynia—three hours away from her home. Only then was she formally—and correctly—diagnosed. First, Katherine tried cutting out certain types of soaps and laundry detergents, wore only white cotton underwear, and avoided certain foods, but to no avail. Skin allergies were not the problem—a dermatologist had ruled out problems such as lichen sclerosus and allergic reactions. Another doctor, a urologist, conducted a cystoscopy for interstitial cystitis, a gastroenterologist did a colonoscopy to rule out inflammatory bowel diseases, and she even went to a rheumatologist to rule out fibromyalgia; Katherine had none of these ailments. Unlike VVS sufferers, Katherine's pain was not provoked. She seemed to experience it without the area being disturbed or touched in any way. Also, as in many women with vulvar dysesthesia, her skin wasn't red, inflamed, or swollen. Yet it continued to hurt. "The pain was affecting me on a daily basis," she explained. "I had extreme stinging, burning, and occasional stabbing feelings in my vulva. When I have flare-ups, it makes daily activities, like sitting, exercising, and of course, sex, nearly impossible."

Today Katherine is seeing some improvement with topical estrogen to help improve elasticity of the tissue at the vaginal opening and intravaginal estrogen to help restore integrity to her pelvic floor musculature. Katherine plans to keep seeing the specialist and stay up-to-date on the latest treatments and studies being done on vulvar dysesthesia. "For my own well-being and daily relief, I have to keep doing whatever it takes to get better," she said recently. She's started a drug called Elavil that helps dull pain, and recently began doing exercises at home that also are starting to help. With combined treatments, her doctors have told Katherine her pain should improve within four months. And after nine months, the average amount of time sufferers spend in treatment, Katherine could even have full relief.

Why Sufferers Need This Book Now

Nearly any woman can be struck by vulvodynia—some are as young as eleven; others are as old as eighty-five. The duration of the disorder can be anywhere from three months to several years. For the lucky patients, the problem eventually goes away by itself. Other women battle with it for years on end. But thankfully, most women find one of many treatment options helpful—and are able to enjoy daily life without pain. They even get back to enjoying fulfilling sex lives.

As is clear from Jordanna's and Katherine's stories, vulvodynia diagnosis and treatment is largely underrecognized—and therefore not well funded for research. While clinical symptoms of vulvodynia are well described, little is known about the origin of these conditions—and there is much yet to learn. That means the road to recovery includes long stretches of medical trial and error. Vulvodynia patients will be told to try this, then something else, then another kind of therapy on top of that. Some courses of treatment will work; some won't. As physicians learn more about vulvodynia, the road to recovery will become less rocky.

Need for Greater Knowledge

When it comes to vulvovaginal pain disorders, there is a true lack of knowledge in the medical community. Women know they have a problem and seek professional advice from their health care providers. Often if practitioners have heard of it at all, they usually don't know what to do about the problem, nor do they have the time and resources it takes to deal with its various aspects. Some may know about it and not believe that it's real.

The message is clear. Many doctors do not yet acknowledge the condition as a real problem with a physical component. Despite a wealth of documented scientific information demonstrating the absence of psychopathology in vulvar pain patients (Meana et al. 1998a), the majority of health care professionals are still slow to embrace and learn about this disorder.

A second problem is this: Most professionals who do recognize and treat vulvodynia don't take an integrated medical approach. Since this disease crosses over many medical subspecialties—such as gynecology, dermatology, urology, gastroenterology, pathology, neurophysiology, immunology, rheumatology, and, of course, psychology and sex therapy—the tendency is for each specialty to only see what they know most about and to use the treatments they are most familiar with. For example, a typical gynecologist may prescribe antifungal creams for yeast infections while a dermatologist may give high-potency topical corticosteroids. Likewise, a urologist may focus on urinary symptoms of urgency and frequency associated with interstitial cystitis; a rheumatologist may focus on muscle aches and pains plus sleep disorders associated with fibromyalgia; immunologists may find evidence of autoimmune problems; endocrinologists may find thyroid problems such as subclinical hypothyroidism; a gastroenterologist may explore nutrition and digestion problems that coexist with vulvodynia such as irritable bowel syndrome; and a neurologist is likely to find nerve problems such as pudendal neuralgia, genital pain caused by nerve damage, or other forms of nerve pain. Meanwhile, a sex therapist is naturally going to deal with the psychological issues. Indeed, there are numerous emotional consequences. (Depression as a result of sexual dysfunction is common.) If the patient's doctors don't coordinate their treatment, they may unintentionally hinder her recovery.

Making the pain go away is one goal. Yet most patients have another goal in mind. Mainly, they want to have intercourse with their partners. They miss, or dream of, having a normal sex life. They apply creams, do exercises, and follow diets for this reason. This points to a third problem: The vast majority of professionals, even gynecologists, are not comfortable discussing sex with their patients.

Sex therapists, as trained mental health practitioners, are likely to search for psychological causes, which often don't exist. Most vulvodynia sufferers *do not* have a history of sexual abuse or sexual dysfunction. What your sex therapist needs to be dealing with is your loss of your sexual self—and helping you get back in touch with that part of your life.

Integrating the knowledge of medical diagnosis and treatment with the principles of sex therapy offers the best possible outcome. Patients need to seek out this treatment and doctors need to provide it. Treating professionals should be comfortable reviewing sexual history, discussing orgasm and clitoral stimulation, masturbation, intercourse duration, libido, physiology of female arousal, anxiety related to sexual pain, and a host of related topics. At first, some patients just want to "fix their genitals." That alone doesn't always work. Patients have to receive sound medical treatment, sometimes including various courses of medication, and emotional support.

This book is written expressly for all women who have ever experienced vulvodynia. The good news is this: The problems don't have to go on as long as Jordanna's and Katherine's. You don't have to suffer while under the care of unknowledgeable doctors. You don't have to live with pain so excruciating that it interrupts your life. Since the medical community is not yet up to speed on vulvodynia, those of you who suspect you have this condition must be in the know. The following pages are filled with the information you need to find care and recovery.

Chapter 1

A Crash Course in Vulvodynia

Not long ago, the popular TV show *Sex in the City* joked that a character with vulvodynia had a depressed vagina. Her fictional female entourage suggested that the woman's vagina might cheer up if they fed it french fries. Some viewers thought it was funny; some did not. But one thing is certain: Vulvodynia can't be solved with a simple french fry. (If only it could be that simple!) The truth is, vulvodynia is no laughing matter—the National Vulvodynia Association estimates that possibly millions of women suffer from chronic vulvar pain at some time in their lives. So while it was great to get the topic on national television, making light of this unfortunate situation isn't funny at all.

For most of those women, the experience has been more of a horror movie than a sitcom. Any sufferer can attest to the complex, painful, often confusing aspects of this disorder. It is difficult to diagnose and even more challenging to treat and manage on a day-to-day basis. Worse still, even when the problem *is* perfectly described by the woman who has it, her doctors may not know enough to diagnose it properly. The sad truth is that most MDs, including many gynecologists, have never heard of vulvodynia. So even though many practitioners have the best intentions, it's no wonder they don't have the first clue when it comes to treatment.

Women usually find out that they have vulvodynia by chance. After seeking help from several different physicians, some luckily stumble onto a doctor who has heard of the condition and can refer them to another practitioner who actually treats it. Other women do the research themselves and end up knowing more than their current doctors. Even more women—it's impossible to know how many exactly—suffer in silence.

VULVA vs. VAGINA: It's important to note that sometimes women confuse the terms **vagina** and **vulva**. The vagina is the canal that extends from the inside of the opening up to the cervix; **vulva** only refers to tissue outside of the vagina including the vaginal opening, the labia, the clitoris, urethra, and the mons pubis. Therefore, vulvodynia only occurs in the vulvar region.

What Is Vulvodynia, Anyway?

If you suspect you have vulvodynia, you need to understand what it means and be familiar with the terms the doctors may use when talking to you. The following are some terms with explanations for most of the problems encompassed under the name vulvodynia.

Vulvodynia is a broad term used to describe any chronic pain in the vulvar area that lasts for at least three months. The term encompasses a variety of conditions with similar symptoms. Before getting into details in later chapters here is a brief introduction to common vulvovaginal problems.

Terms You Should Know

Vulvodynia. Chronic vulvar itching, burning, and pain that causes physical, sexual, and psychological distress. This term means pain in the vulva and is a description of several symptoms—not a formal diagnosis. The word comes from the Greek term for pain, which is *odynia*. "Vulv" indicates the location of the pain, which in this case is the vulva, the external area of the genitalia. Vulvar pain may be due to many causes, including infections, benign skin conditions, hormone depletion, trauma, nerve damage, and, rarely, precancerous or malignant conditions. All of the above can contribute to vulvodynia. Note: A similar syndrome occurs in males called prostatodynia or scrotodynia, in which certain areas of the male genitalia are afflicted with pain and discomfort.

Dysesthetic vulvodynia. The word *dysesthesia* means "altered sensation." Dysesthetic vulvodynia includes symptoms of chronic or intermittent burning, stinging, itching, rawness, and irritation in the vulva. The discomfort varies and is unprovoked, meaning it can occur without being touched or disturbed in any way. A light touch with a wisp of cotton may feel like scraping or stabbing. The diagnosis is given to vulvar pain patients who have this sensory dysfunction and/or unprovoked pain.

Vulvar vestibulitis. Discomfort or pain that is located only on the vulvar vestibule, which is the shiny mucous tissue surrounding the vaginal opening inside the "lips" of the vulva. Patients often describe this condition as a sharp stabbing or cutting sensation. Pain is always worse with provocation, such as with intercourse (known as *introital dyspareunia*) or tampon insertion. In some patients, pain occurs from wearing tight clothing, prolonged sitting, or such physical activities as bicycling or horseback riding. Note: Vestibulitis also has been called *vestibulodynia, focal vulvar dysesthesia, vulvar vestibulitis syndrome*, and *vestibular adenitis*. Presently, *vulvar vestibulitis* syndrome (VVS) remains the most common term used by members of the International Society for the Study of Vulvovaginal Disease (ISSVD).

For the remainder of this book, we'll use the term *vestibulitis*, or VVS. (Note: Some new proposed classifications for vulvar pain being contemplated by the ISSVD consider both vestibulitis and vulvodynia to be vulvar dysesthesia, and discriminate between generalized, unprovoked dysesthesia (including most patients with dysesthetic, or essential, vulvodynia) and focal, provoked (consistent with pure vestibulitis) vulvar dysesthesia. While these may be more specific descriptions and more consistent with the terms used in pain literature and pathology classification systems, they are too unwieldy to be practical. So we will use the terms *vulvodynia* and *vestibulitis*.)

Dyspareunia. Pain during intercourse due to any cause. Vulvodynia causes much difficulty with intercourse—that is, if the woman is able to have it at all. Note that introital dyspareunia, which is pain at the opening of the vagina during attempted penetration, is different than deep dyspareunia, which refers to discomfort deep inside the vagina during thrusting. Introital dyspareunia is a key symptom of vulvar vestibulitis problems. Deep dyspareunia is most often associated with other issues such as endometriosis, uterine fibroids, or bladder and bowel hypersensitivity.

Pudendal neuralgia. Pain in the area served by the pudendal nerves. Neuralgia means pain caused by nerve damage or dysfunction, and in this case, the word refers to pain arising from the pudendal nerve, the only pelvic nerve with both sensory and motor function. The discomfort of pudendal neuralgia usually follows the pathway of the pudendal nerve, which serves the entire vulvar area, including the clitoris and mons pubis, the hair-bearing region of the vulva. Pain can occur anywhere in the vulva or perineum including the pubic, perianal, and clitoral area.

Perineal pain syndrome. Consists of irritation or pain in the perineum, the external area from the bottom of the vaginal opening down to the anal opening. This term is truly as broad as vulvodynia because it encompasses many types of pain in that region.

The difference between the generic term *vulvodynia* and the more specific words *dysesthetic vulvodynia* and *vestibulitis* should now be clearer. Just to review, with dysesthetic vulvodynia, pain can be located anywhere in the vulva and may even extend beyond the vulva into the perineum or even onto the thighs. Vestibulitis is localized in the vulvar vestibule and occurs when provoked by clothing, sitting, vigorous activity, or penetration. Women say vestibulitis feels like a stabbing, sharp sensation in that area, causing acute pain. Dysesthetic vulvodynia, on the other hand, is more diffuse and can occur anywhere in the vulvar region, and is chronic or recurrent. It occurs spontaneously, without provocation and feels more like burning. Pudendal neuralgia is a form of vulvodynia in which pain is experienced at the endings of the sensory branches of the pudendal nerve and may more often cause pain in the anterior vulvar area, near the urethra, clitoris, and mons pubis.

Vulvovaginal Anatomy 101

It's nearly impossible to understand vulvar disorders and their origins without full comprehension of the anatomy of the vulva and the vagina. It's all too common for women to be extremely unfamiliar with their own genitals. In fact, most females have not even looked at or examined their own vulvas with a hand mirror. It is important that you do so. Some women won't be bothered a bit by this exercise—others may be shy at first. Both reactions are healthy and normal. Just make sure you do your own exam in the next few weeks. Not only will you know exactly where your pain exists and how to describe it; but being able to visualize where everything is will help you understand the complicated medical explanations your doctors will give you. Be aware that vulvas are like faces, no two are exactly alike. The shape and size of the labia minora are especially variable in normal women. To get an idea of the range of normal appearances, see Betty Dodson's book *Sex for One* (1996). Your body is yours, and you'll benefit the most from understanding it. Take a look at figures 1 and 2 and review the medical terms for your vulvar anatomy.

Points of Reference

Anus. The opening of the rectum located between the buttocks.

Bartholin's glands. Located on either side of the vaginal opening just inside the skin. (Locate them by thinking of the vestibule as a clock face with the clitoris resting at twelve o'clock. Bartholin's glands are located at four and eight o'clock.) They produce small amounts of lubricating fluid that keeps the inner labia moist when you are sexually aroused. The production can go down with inflammation or with age. Cysts can occur in this location and cause pain with sitting or attempts to use tampons or have intercourse.

Clitoris. This is a small oval-shaped body of spongy tissue located at top of the labia minora and covered by the clitoral hood, a flap of skin located just above the clitoris that protects it. It is highly sexually sensitive. During sexual excitement, the clitoris may extend and the hood retract to make the clitoris more accessible.

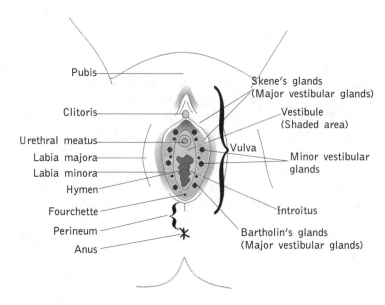

Figure 1. The external female genitals, known as the vulva, including the pubis, clitoris, urethral opening, labia majora, labia minora, vulvar vestibule, and vaginal opening (introitus).

Labia majora. These are the outer, larger lips of the vulva. They are made of fatty pads of tissue that wrap around the vulva from the mons veneris to the perineum. They are usually covered with pubic hair and contain many oil and sweat glands.

Labia minora. These are the inner, smaller lips of the vulva. They are the thin stretches of tissue within the labia majora that protect the vagina, urethra, and clitoris. They can vary in size from woman to woman and are sensitive to touch and pressure.

Mons veneris. This is the fatty pad of tissue that covers the pubic bone. It is below the abdomen but above the labia. It is in the area where the pubic hairline starts. The mons is sexually sensitive and protects the pubic bone during the thrusting of intercourse. (*Mons veneris* is the Latin for "hill of Venus," the Roman goddess of love.)

Perineum. The short stretch of skin starting at the bottom of the vulva and extending to the anus.

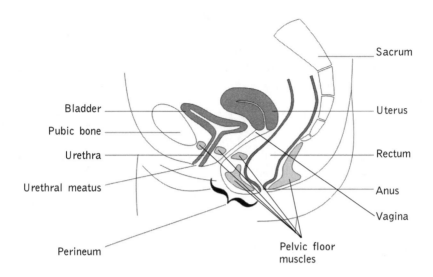

Bladder

Pubic bone

Urethra

Urethral meatus

Perineum

Sacrum

Uterus

Rectum

Anus

Vagina

Pelvic floor
muscles

Figure 2. A side view of the female pelvis showing the relationship of the pelvic floor muscles to the bladder, urethra, vagina, and rectum.

Skene's glands. They are also known as the periurethral glands, and appear as a small indentation on either side of the urethral meatus, the opening where urine comes out. These glands are thought to be of the same tissue origin as the male prostate glands. (In some women who "ejaculate" during extreme sexual excitement, this is where the fluid probably comes from.)

Urethra. This is located just below the clitoris. It is a passage for urine that is connected to the bladder and does not serve reproductive functions.

Vagina. This is the opening that extends into your body to your cervix. It serves as the receptacle for the penis during sexual intercourse, and is the birth canal during labor. The average vagina is three inches long and the canal expands during sexual arousal and childbirth.

Vestibule. The innermost area of the vulva, closest to the vaginal entrance, just outside the hymen. The vestibule surrounds the vaginal entrance (known as the introitus), and is shiny, hairless tissue that is, in fact, a mucous lining and not skin. This oval-shaped area extends side to side from the inner aspects of the labia minora to the vaginal opening, and front to back from the underside of the clitoris to the fourchette (just above the perineum, which is the web of skin between the vagina and anus). The vestibule includes the urethral and vaginal openings as well as the openings of the major and minor vestibular glands, which are located in the groove at the base of the hymen (see figure 1).

Vulva. The term refers to the external female genital organs including the labia majora, labia minora, vestibule, clitoris, urethra, and hymenal ring.

What Sufferers Can Expect

Vulvar pain rears its head in many different ways and may be hard for women to describe. One woman may feel burning or aching all over and another may be bothered by intermittent itching sensations. Still other women may only complain of pain when a certain area is touched during activities such as sexual intercourse, tampon insertion, or even routine gynecological exams. The pain can be something the sufferer is all too used to—many women have had it since the first time they tried to insert a tampon. But for others, the onset of pain may arrive without warning. They may develop it—in their late teens or not until their sixties. In some cases, experts believe the onset of vulvodynia is associated with some form of vulvar irritation or trauma such as recurrent vaginal infections. It could be triggered by episodes of yeast infections, infection by the herpes virus or the human papilloma virus (HPV), the trauma of childbirth, onset of menopause or other hormonal changes, or certain diseases or therapeutic procedures including surgery.

Because vulvar pain symptoms are most often associated with the above forms of vulvar irritation, it is not known whether vulvodynia is caused by these irritants or traumatic events themselves, if it is caused by the treatments given for these ailments (such as topical antifungals for yeast), or if it's caused by a patient's own tendency for vulvar irritation. It may be due to a natural response—as the woman's body fights the presumed cause of pain, pelvic muscle spasms deprive the genitals of proper blood flow. It may also have to do with the sufferer's threshold of sensation or the number of nerve endings she has. Usually, there is not a single phenomenon responsible for vulvodynia. Instead, a series of events that act on a healthy but irritation-prone vulva seem to have a cumulative effect. Infections, treatments, and surgeries may exacerbate vulvar symptoms, causing a full-blown case of vulvodynia.

Vulvodynia can be classified as either organic (existing from a known cause) or essential (of unknown origin). In traditional medicine, essential (also called idiopathic or functional) conditions are diagnosed by ruling out all other known causes of pain, such as infections and diseases. Basically, when practitioners can't find the source of a problem, they deem it "essential." (Unfortunately, even some very sympathetic physicians frequently take the next, often unwarranted, step of assuming that because essential disorders can't be explained, they must be psychological in origin. This line of thinking is precisely why a doctor may tell a patient that her vulvar problems are all in her head. From the doctor's perspective, here is a patient whose only symptoms are self-reports of vulvar and sexual pain and possibly vaginal discharge that may or may not be due to yeast. Because of her pain and its effects on her life, she is probably in a state of emotional distress. Yet the doctor can't find anything wrong, and certainly the patient's problem isn't life threatening. So, the physician deems her pain of psychological origin, sometimes referred to as "psychogenic vulvar pain." Not only does this deprive patients of some useful treatment options, it labels them as being somehow psychologically "unstable" or less credible—and their problems less worthy of serious investigation. This can result in further suffering.

The whole experience of not knowing what's wrong can be extremely frustrating. And it makes diagnosis much more difficult for doctors who aren't experienced in treating vulvodynia.

This is why many doctors simply don't treat the condition, and have little interest in doing so. Physicians are trained to diagnose problems and treat them with medication, therapy, or surgery. Most of the time, vulvodynia is clearly difficult to diagnose. Once it is named, patients often need a combination of treatments—and even those may not work. There is no known miracle cure for sufferers. Vulvodynia treatment is incredibly time-consuming for doctors, which may be one reason they shy away from the problem. Often, distraught, demanding patients who are eager for answers make the doctor's job even more difficult.

Why Diagnosis Is So Difficult

It's common for patients to feel swelling, irritation, and discharge with vulvodynia. Often, women head to the doctor thinking they have yeast or urinary tract infections. Patients ask (some beg) for the usual prescriptions. Likewise, medical professionals who are less familiar with vulvodynia will tend to prescribe patients antifungals to fight yeast and antibiotics to ward off bad bladder bacteria. Often medications are given even if urinalysis and microscopic vaginal fluid examination does not confirm the presence of yeast or bacteria. That's because the patients are insisting that yeast and/or urinary tract infection symptoms exist (but discomfort is actually due to vulvodynia). Doctors prescribe medicine because they just don't know what else to do. Treating symptoms is part of their job. Sometimes, everyone gets lucky and the medication "works," or time passes and the pain goes away spontaneously. More often, however, none of these treatments work, or a doctor will conduct more sophisticated laboratory tests that rule out yeast and urinary tract infections. When the symptoms persist, an evaluation for vulvodynia is needed.

Now, there is another problem with the average, well-meaning gynecologist who doesn't specialize in these problems. Just because he or she takes a vaginal swab of a patient's secretions, looks at it under a microscope, and says "no yeast" doesn't always mean the doctor is correct. Many gynecologists don't specialize in infectious disease and may not recognize the less common forms of candida. (Most yeast infections are caused by easily identifiable Candida albicans. Still, there are many other candida fungi that can cause problems.) Different forms of yeast or bacteria are sensitive to different antifungals or antibiotics—and they require different prescriptions and durations than the average albican yeast infection does. A gynecologist may therefore try many more courses of treatment before finding an effective one, and the treatments themselves can also be irritating to sensitive genital tissue.

Similarly, gynecologists don't routinely tell patients if they see anything out of the ordinary on the vulva. They may be reluctant to make patients more self-conscious or embarrassed than they already are during an exam. Also, the appearance of vulvar tissue—even in symptom-free patients—varies greatly. Doctors are taught to look for signs of cancer—a serious, life-threatening illness—so they may not think that non-threatening changes, like the ones seen in patients who complain of vulvar pain, are anything to be concerned about. Some are not. But some changes, which result from hormone loss, laser treatments, or other treatments for HPV, vulvar dermatoses, and other ailments, *are* big deals—especially for sensitive patients who are in pain. A woman could have damaged tissue from any of the above, and the doctor may not recognize it or choose to mention it. Unless a problem or irregularity is noticed, it won't be treated.

Is It Dysesthetic Vulvodynia?

Recurrent rawness, itching, and burning anywhere from the mons pubis to the anus points to dysesthetic vulvodynia, especially if the symptoms are far worse than the somewhat healthy appearance of the vulva would suggest. If you can't seem to pinpoint your pain, but it keeps coming back, this could possibly be your problem. Usually women with this type of vulvodynia have constant pain with brief periods of unexplained relief. Their symptoms in particular may mimic the ones seen in bladder infections. For example, they may have to urinate frequently, urgently, and they experience pain when urinating. Yet, there are no unfriendly bacteria in their urine causing problems.

Most annoyingly, the pain just won't go away. Some women have pain when they try to have intercourse (dyspareunia); some do not have additional trouble with sex. But who wants to have sex when there's nonstop burning? Sex isn't their main issue—the constant pain is. That becomes the most pressing problem. Some experts believe the cause of vulvar dysesthesia is neuropathic, meaning that the nervous system is the culprit. It could be a result of nerve trauma, stretching, inflammation, pressure on nerves from discs, or scars from surgical incisions. Or possibly, the muscles and joints are damaged or stressed, and nerves are likewise negatively affected. Spinal problems, such as ruptured discs or scarring, may also lead to vulvar dysesthesia.

Most women who are diagnosed with dysesthetic vulvodynia, which includes pudendal neuralgia and perineal pain sufferers, fit certain characteristics. A recent study found that the typical patient is about forty years old, and more than half were married (Sadownik 2000). Also, 55 percent had other chronic health conditions, such as allergies or back pain. Regardless of socioeconomic factors, most patients were Caucasian. For unknown reasons, African-American women as a group are the least likely to report vulvar dysesthesia, or any other type of vulvodynia.

Once the pain is diagnosed, you can expect to feel a huge sense of relief. Now at least you know you don't have cancer or anything life-threatening. You do, however, have quite a journey ahead of you. First, most doctors advise women with vulvar dysesthesia to avoid dyes, chemicals, fragrances, and other chemicals that cause irritation. Patients are also advised to wear only white cotton underwear and loose-fitting clothing. Mini- and maxipads are also not good ideas because they rub against and irritate the affected areas. As for treatment options, expect a combination of drugs. You may be given topical local anesthetics, such as lidocaine, to help relieve the pain briefly during periods of flare-up or for use with attempted intercourse. The other common treatment is tricyclic antidepressants, usually amitriptyline or nortriptyline.

Antidepressants have been shown to block nerve pain, and may help to reduce or eliminate vulvar pain. Occasionally, early side effects may need to be tolerated, such as drowsiness, dryness, and weight gain, but these often subside over time. Also, drug dosages may need to be adjusted upwards until they work, and it may be up to three months before they take full effect.

If after three months of taking correct dosages, you still haven't seen any improvement in your pain, doctors may try anticonvulsants such as gabapentin (commonly called Neurontin), dilantin, or carbamazepine, which help nerves tolerate more stimulation before firing off pain signals. Another option is a pelvic floor muscle evaluation by surface electromyography (sEMG). An sEMG of your pelvic floor muscles is similar to an electrocardiogram, or EKG, of your heart muscle. This technology can detect muscle abnormalities that play a role in pain mechanisms (Glazer, Rodke, et al. 1995). Later your doctor may prescribe neuromuscular rehabilitation of the pelvic floor, using biofeedback. This treatment involves an exercise regimen aimed at correcting the muscle abnormality. You exercise the pelvic floor muscles daily using a small tampon-like device inserted in the vagina and connected to a device that allows them to "see" the activity of the muscles as they exercise. This can help restore the pelvic floor muscles back to a healthy condition. Still another treatment is the use of dilators, which is common and noninvasive. These are medical devices that gradually stretch the vaginal circumference. You can do this at home, at your own pace, in order to become comfortable with your ability to touch and control entry to your own vagina. This makes exams and intercourse more physically comfortable later on. (For more details on your treatment options, see chapter 4.)

Is It Vestibulitis?

According to recent estimates, up to 15 percent of the female population currently suffers from vulvar vestibulitis (Denbow and Byrne 1998). It is characterized by localized, consistent pain in the vulvar vestibule. Often, the area turns red (doctors call this erythema) and becomes swollen. Sometimes, not always, it can be detected with a hand mirror. Reddish, swollen tissue is often *not* present (Bergeron et al. 1994). Nonetheless, it is definitely worth looking for, as it sometimes is associated with other conditions. In most patients, the redness and/or inflammation does not occur until the area is touched. It may occur as a result of penile penetration, from wearing tight clothing, during tampon insertion and removal, or when exams are performed. (Deeper pains—in the vagina and pelvis—are associated with different problems such as endometriosis, uterine fibroids, and urinary or bowel disorders such as interstitial cystitis or irritable bowel syndrome.) Basically any sensitivity in the organs of the lower pelvic region including bowel, bladder, and uterus can lead to pain with thrusting. While these disorders may coexist with vestibulitis, they are not necessarily part of the disorder.

Since the vestibule includes the introitus or vaginal opening, vestibulitis is often associated with pain during intercourse. Some women with vestibulitis can tolerate sex, many cannot. Some have had dyspareunia since their first sexual experience, in which case it's called *primary*. Others have *secondary* dyspareunia that developed after having years of normal, pain-free sexual activity. A major complaint of women with vestibulitis is the damage it does to their sexuality. Many can't engage in intercourse at all.

What Causes It?

Why certain women end up with this disorder remains a mystery, though many theories exist. For years vestibulitis was supposedly caused by candida, or yeast infections. But more recent studies have shown that vestibulitis patients don't have more yeast in their vaginas than other women (Bazin et al. 1994). Often, women mistake their vestibulitis symptoms—itching and burning—for yeast infections.

Doctors usually do the same and antifungals are prescribed. The irritation doesn't go away, and it's possible that the antifungals aggravate the area (Sobel et al. 1998). HPV was also considered a cause of vestibulitis (Marinoff and Turner 1992), but that thinking is waning. Newer studies have shown that HPV is rarely found in the vestibule (Goetsch 1999), and subtypes of HPV all fail to demonstrate a correlation with vestibulitis (Wilkinson et al. 1993).

Common treatments for HPV, such as trichloroacetic acid (TCA) and laser surgery for removing warts, do seem to irritate the vestibular area further. One researcher (Solomons, Melmed, and Heiter 1991) has presented a case study suggesting a relationship between urinary oxalates and vestibulitis. Another researcher (Baggish, Sze, and Johnson 1997) has demonstrated no difference in twenty-four urinary oxalate excretions in vestibulitis patients as compared to matched controls. Recent studies (Glazer et al. 1998) have demonstrated that vestibulitis patients show significantly different pelvic floor muscle sEMG tracings than normal, but it is not known if these muscle dysfunctions exist before the symptoms and predispose patients to this condition or if this muscle dysfunction occurs as a result of the pain syndrome and then maintains it. An increase in psychiatric problems is not associated with vestibulitis (Meana et al. 1998b); this disorder is not considered to be psychogenic.

Perhaps the most exciting new data relating to vestibulitis comes out of recent laboratory research suggesting that vestibulitis pain is *nociceptive*, that is, it arises from persistent inflammatory damage to tissue. Certain women may be genetically predisposed to make more chemicals that increase or cause inflammation (Witkin et al. 2000). In this theory, vulvar irritations cause the release of certain chemicals (cytokines), which sensitize nerve endings, causing normal touch to be experienced as pain (a condition called *allodynia*). Supporting this theory is recent research showing an increase in the number of nerve fibers in the vulvar vestibule of vestibulitis patients (Bohm-Starke et al. 1998). Further support comes from studies showing that vestibular tissue samples of vestibulitis sufferers have higher levels of natural substances that promote inflammation (Slone et al. 1999).

How Is It Diagnosed?

Vestibulitis is a diagnosis of exclusion. That means vaginal infections such as yeast, bacteria, and virus are first ruled out; then doctors have to make sure that dermatological problems such as vulvar dermatitis, allergic reactions, lichen simplex chronicus, lichen sclerosus, lichen planus, and other problems aren't present, or that these problems have been recognized and treated before a final diagnosis. Many other similar diseases must also be considered. Once a doctor knows for sure that no other problem is active—yet the irritation is still there—vestibulitis can finally be diagnosed.

The typical sufferer is usually younger than a vulvar dysesthesia patient. The average age is thirty-two, but women in their twenties and even teens are also frequently diagnosed. Again, Caucasian women have vestibulitis more than any other racial group (Marinoff and Turner 1992). The problem doesn't seem affected by socioeconomic status (Neill and Ridley 1999).

The course of treatment is similar to that of vulvar dysesthesia. First, dyes, fragrances, soaps, and tight clothes should be eliminated. Topical estrogen such as estradiol cream may help improve the tender tissue. Then tricyclic antidepressants, such as amitriptyline, may be prescribed for their pain-blocking qualities. Some women have great success on them, but many do not. The next step is to try anticonvulsants, such as gabapentin (Neurontin). The use of dilators is often prescribed to desensitize and stretch the tissue of the vestibule. Electromyographic biofeedback has also proved helpful (Glazer et al. 1995). Treatment typically progresses from less to more invasive procedures. A next step often includes vulvar injections of interferon to boost immune system function in patients who test positive for HPV. Finally, there are many different forms of surgery from Bartholin's gland removal to full vestibulectomy with perineoplasty and vaginal advancement. Surgery has proven extremely successful. Of course, with surgery, there is a risk of creating tender scar tissue as well. That is why women usually try everything else before resorting to surgical procedures.

How Other Ailments Come into Play

Many women (but not all, of course) with vulvar pain have other genital problems. According to an extensive, albeit not formally scientific, Web site survey of 2,473 women with vulvodynia done by Howard Glazer, a large percent of sufferers have coexisting conditions. They are dealing with many issues besides vulvodynia. (See chapter 2 for full details.) A widely accepted theory is that women with vulvodynia have a predisposition for inflammation. Some women even lack the gene, called the polymorphism gene, which helps inflamed skin get back to normal (Witkin, Gerber, and Ledger 2002). But whether that gene is present or not, the ability to block inflammation seems out of whack in most patients with vulvodynia. Researchers are currently looking more deeply into this problem for definitive answers. Right now, there aren't many. But this inability to attack and heal inflammation may help explain why many of the following conditions coexist with vulvodynia.

Associated Disorders

Fibromyalgia, a condition with symptoms of widespread pain, tenderness, fatigue, and exhaustion, afflicts many women with vulvovaginal pain. Experts don't know how fibromyalgia is related to essential vulvar pain (of an unknown cause), but they do know that fibromyalgia and vulvodynia often coexist. Similarly, interstitial cystitis, an inflammation of the bladder lining, is associated with vulvodynia. Chronic migraines are also associated. Irritable bowel syndrome is another condition affecting many vulvar pain sufferers and involves a dysfunction in gut activity possibly related to a hyperactive response to input from the nervous system. Other autoimmune or inflammatory disorders commonly seen are lupus (a systemic disease that involves any part or organ of the body), sarcoidosis (another systemic disease), or Hashimoto's thyroiditis (a chronic inflammatory condition resulting in thyroid malfunction).

Dermographism

Dermographism is a condition in which people wheal, or welt up, after pressure is put on the skin. It is caused by the release of inflammatory chemicals such as histamines, which causes small blood vessels to leak, resulting in tissue swelling. It is thought that this process of histamine inflammation and blood vessel leakage may also be going on in the vulvar vestibule. Some vestibulitis sufferers don't have noticeable redness until after they are examined or touched in the vestibule. This may be a form of dermographism. Again, the link to inflammatory trouble could be the underlying problem—and the reason why dermographism often coexists with vestibulitis.

Lichen Sclerosus

Lichen sclerosus is a disorder that is sometimes associated with vulvodynia. It causes the skin to thin and become pale and less elastic, and can occur in other areas of the body besides the vulvar region. Lichen sclerosus is most commonly seen in post-menopausal women, but also in women as young as their teens and even in young children. There is a thinning of the upper dermis or layer of skin and inflammation in the dermis below. Some women with lichen sclerosus suffer constant burning and itching in the vestibular area. Sufferers' tight, thin vulvar skin resists the stretching efforts of tampons, fingers, the penis, or a speculum. Sometimes the skin is so thin that the top layer is easily rubbed off or cracked, especially during intercourse. This is, of course, painful when it occurs. But many women have mild cases and few symptoms, so they may not know they have it. This condition can coexist with essential vulvodynia. It is therefore important to rule it out or treat it. Another, similar condition that includes the symptoms of itching and burning is *lichen planus*. This is an autoimmune, inflammatory skin disease that can affect all areas of the skin as well as the lining of the mouth and genitalia.

Sexually Transmitted Diseases

Herpes, human papilloma virus (sometimes called genital warts), and other sexually transmitted diseases can cause symptoms of burning, itching, and redness. Some patients may think they've contracted an STD when they haven't. Others may have an autoimmune disorder along with vulvodynia. And some research indicates that the irritation caused by these disorders can trigger vulvodynia.

Myths and Misconceptions About Vulvodynia

Now that you have some basic information about the condition, it's important to understand a few of the common misconceptions about vulvodynia. The following list of facts debunks some popularly held myths.

1. **Fact: Vulvodynia is not a sexually transmitted disease.** Many women worry that they can get it or give it to partners. They absolutely cannot. They also cannot get it from a partner. It is not a contagious condition in any way. (An exception: If you've tested positive for HPV or herpes. These STDs can exacerbate the symptoms of vulvodynia.)

2. **Fact: Having vulvodynia does not cause cancer or increase your risks of getting it.** Vulvodynia has nothing to do with cancer. It is important to note, however, that some forms of cancer can cause vulvar pain that can mimic symptoms of vulvodynia. So getting checked out is always important. Otherwise, cancer and essential forms of vulvodynia have nothing to do with each other in cause or effect.

3. **Fact: Vulvodynia is not in women's heads.** Psychological studies show that in spite of the emotional reactivity and depression and anxiety that may result from suffering vulvar pain, vulvodynia patients are not different from the normal population (Meana et al. 1998b). The emotional reaction we see is usually an appropriate reaction to pain. (That doesn't mean that psychopathology can't coexist with vulvodynia. But vulvodynia sufferers are no more likely to have underlying psychiatric problems than the population at large.) It is clear that vulvodynia can cause psychological problems, even after pain is greatly reduced or eliminated. Due to the loss of their sexual selves, another painful aspect of vulvodynia, patients may need therapy for full recovery.

4. **Fact: Vulvodynia is not correlated with a higher incidence of past sexual abuse.** There is no higher incidence of sexual abuse in women with vulvodynia than there is in the population at large (Meana et al. 1998b). Sexual abuse is

probably more common than most people know, however. If you have been abused, it is important to find a therapist to help you recover; those emotional scars can further interfere with your recovery from vulvodynia.

5. **Fact: Vulvodynia is often associated with a history of vaginal yeast infections, HPV, and urinary tract infections.** The above problems coexist with vulvodynia for many women—but not all of them. (Some researchers believe recurrent vaginal infections trigger long-term vulvodynia.) Careful evaluation is needed because various vulvar infections often mimic vulvodynia. You don't want to be treated for a yeast infection if you don't really have one! It won't help you get relief from true vulvodynia. Also, some women develop reactions to creams over time, so it may even make your vulvodynia worse. (On the other hand, vulvodynia won't keep you from getting a yeast or bladder infection. So if your symptoms are worse than usual, it is worth checking for other problems.)

6. **Fact: With proper treatment, sufferers can live normal, healthy lives that include good sex.** Again, the road to recovery can be long. But as thousands of women who no longer experience vulvar pain can attest, it doesn't have to last forever. You can—and will—get better once you're armed with knowledge and the proper treatments.

Chapter 2

Could You Have Vulvodynia?

If you're reading this book, you probably think you have some form of vulvodynia (or perhaps you have a loved one who does). The following quiz will help you determine if you're suffering from the disorder. Bear in mind that although our quiz can give you a good indication of your own condition, it should not be substituted for a knowledgeable doctor's opinion. Nor should it keep you from getting a proper diagnosis from a qualified medical care professional. However, you can take the results of this quiz to your doctor. They are sure to provide him or her with valuable insight.

Self-Test: Find Out If You Are a Likely Sufferer

Please answer yes or no to the following questions:

Part I: Your Vulvodynia Profile

1. Have you been treated for various vaginal infections (yeast, urinary tract, etc.), but still had pain after the treatments were completed?

2. Have you had recurring cycles of urinary tract and yeast infections that seem to come one after another?

3. Has this ever happened to you? You go into the doctor's office complaining of a vaginal infection, yet when tests are run, the physician can't find signs of infection or anything else that is wrong.

4. Did your symptoms start after a series of yeast, bacterial, or urinary tract infections, or after genital trauma such as pelvic surgery or a fall?

5. Do you suffer from allergies or skin conditions?

6. Have you ever been diagnosed with interstitial cystitis, irritable bowel syndrome, fibromyalgia, or any autoimmune or inflammatory disorder?

7. Have you experienced a decline in your usual level of sexual interest, frequency, or pleasure?

8. Are you depressed or suffering from psychological distress?

If you answered yes to at least four of the above questions, you match the profile of a typical vulvodynia sufferer. For an even more specific profile, answer yes or no to the following statements.

Part II: Could You Have Vestibulitis?

1. Is discomfort only present when the vulva is touched (by tight clothing, tampon use, or during penetration)?

2. Is the pain usually very near the vaginal opening?

3. Is the pain usually localized in the same spot or spots within this area?

If you answered yes to at least two of these questions, you probably have the condition known as vestibulitis. If you answered no to at least two of the above questions, read on. You may have another form of vulvodynia.

Part III: Could You Have Dysesthetic Vulvodynia?

1. Is your vulvar pain present most or all of the time, seemingly appearing for no apparent reason?

2. Have you suffered a back injury or a straddle injury while biking, working out, or horseback riding?

3. Do you have chronic back pain?

4. Would you describe the pain as a diffuse, burning sensation? (It can be located on any part of your vulva.)

5. Are you age 35 or older?

6. When touched, is the feeling you get strange? (Does a cotton swab feel like a needle? Does a light touch feel like sandpaper?)

If you answered yes to at least three of these questions, you probably have the condition known as dysesthetic vulvodynia.

(Note: While unusual, it is possible to have both vestibulitis and dysesthetic vulvodynia simultaneously.)

Defining the Experience of Vulvodynia

For the last three years, coauthor Howard Glazer has posted a survey on his informational Web site, www.vulvodynia.com. The purpose was to collect data to better understand sufferers' lives. He hoped to understand his own patients better—which has definitely been the result.

Although this method of collecting survey information does not meet scientific standards, the information that presented itself is still interesting and valuable. For a body of research to be considered scientifically valid, researchers must ask questions from a very large number of randomly selected people. In other words, a significant segment of the vulvodynia sufferer population would first need to be identified, and then a sample of that population would be randomly selected and questioned. Glazer was unable to take such complex, precise measures, but instead, encouraged the thousands of women who visited his informational Web site to answer a lengthy questionnaire. Respondents who wanted to be involved did so voluntarily. In fact, because so many women—more than two thousand—answered the questionnaire, his study became more revealing and important than he had imagined. So while the data does not reach the level of scientific standards, it does accurately represent the feelings and experiences of a specific sample of sufferers. Their answers can't be blanket statements for the vulvar pain population as a whole, but they do represent the self-selected group of women who participated.

Most interestingly, the women who participated have helped to provide first-ever details about the lives and habits of typical sufferers. The survey also points out specific traits that vulvar pain patients have in common. Some of the information is surprising. For example, a large majority of sufferers wear glasses or contacts. While more thorough research needs to be conducted, the possible association between vision problems and vulvar pain is interesting.

The information gleaned from the survey also coincides with previous vulvodynia research and literature. In some areas, the study takes well-documented ideas about vulvodynia and takes them a step further. Glazer has also looked at medical history, details of sexual functioning, and self-reports of the typical treatments for vulvodynia and their effectiveness. In short, the study reveals what it feels like to be a sufferer.

Many patients ask the same question: "Do other women say they've felt the same way?" This survey's results validate their situations and daily feelings. If nothing else, it lets them know they are not alone.

The Survey

So, who participated? As this book went to press, 2,473 women, all who have some form of vulvodynia, filled out the questionnaire of their own accord after visiting the Web site www.vulvodynia.com. There were 168 questions total, and the survey took respondents approximately forty minutes to complete. What follows are the most revealing and interesting questions and answers.

The Typical Sufferer

- Age: Most vulvar pain patients were between the ages of twenty-one and thirty-four (57 percent), and a secondary group was between the ages thirty-five and fifty (43 percent).

- Relationship status: The vast majority of patients were married or living with a partner (73 percent).

- Education: Most had an above average level of education (59 percent completed college).

- Work: Most sufferers (63 percent) indicated professional, managerial occupations.

- Money: Their socioeconomic status was higher than average; 62 percent reported incomes greater than $50,000 annually.

- Race: An overwhelming 90 percent of patients were Caucasian, while less than 1 percent were of African origin.

What it all means. There is a bimodal or double-peaked distribution of age, meaning that most respondents were ages twenty-one to thirty-four, with the secondary age between thirty-five and fifty. Most likely, the former group represents primarily vestibulitis patients, and the second group represents primarily dysesthetic vulvodynia patients.

Somewhat surprisingly, most of these women had boyfriends or partners. This is a positive finding that may mean vulvar pain doesn't necessarily lead to breakdowns in intimate relationships. (However, it can change the nature of them, as sexual intercourse often becomes impossible.)

The higher levels of socioeconomic, education, and occupation status is consistent with previous studies. Why? Unfortunately, it's probably because educated women with access to money for medical care are the most likely to pursue the best, most specialized medical treatments (or at least to use the Internet).

Caucasian women reported more vulvar pain than any other ethnic group. African-American women rarely report these conditions. Researchers aren't sure why this is true, though it has been commonly observed by many of our colleagues in the International Society for the Study of Vulvovaginal Disease, who practice and teach in various medical settings where women of various races and incomes are seen. Other dark-skinned ethnic groups, such as Indians, do report chronic vulvar pain syndromes.

Her Female Functioning

Menstruation. Most women with these conditions were between the ages of twelve to fourteen when they got their first periods (85 percent). A high majority of them were experiencing regular periods at the time they completed the survey (80 percent) and did not have out-of-the-ordinary menstrual pain (81 percent). Most didn't have mid-cycle bleeding (88 percent). Respondents used pads and tampons almost equally (51 percent preferred pads, 49 percent tampons). And many of them (44 percent) used oral contraceptives. This data tells us that most vulvar pain patients have normal menstrual function. Plus, vulvar pain does not appear to be affected by a woman's choice of pads versus tampons.

Childbearing. The women were evenly split—half had never been pregnant and half have had at least one pregnancy. For those who had experienced pregnancy, less than 30 percent had miscarriages or abortions. In the women who delivered children, 70 percent had vaginal deliveries and 30 percent delivered by C-sections. As for women who experienced vaginal deliveries, 2 percent reported that forceps were used, 53 percent reported episiotomies, and 38 percent reported "tearing" during delivery. The good news: Pregnant vulvodynia patients do not have abortions or miscarriages more often than other women; the Cesarean section rate may be somewhat higher due to patient preference or due to the well-intentioned recommendation of doctors who wish to avoid adding a tender episiotomy scar to the patient's problems. Vulvar patients who experienced vaginal deliveries report no more frequent use of forceps or episiotomies than the population at large.

Sex. Most women had their first sexual intercourse between the ages of fourteen to nineteen (70 percent). Half of the women reported four or fewer sexual partners and half had five or more. The vast majority (90 percent) had never been sexually abused—not as children or adults. Most had never had a sexually transmitted disease (77 percent). But of the 23 percent of women who have had an STD, most of them reported that they have been diagnosed as having HPV (86 percent).

The age at which patients first had intercourse is no different from that of the population at large. Their number of sexual partners is also comparable to average women. So sexual activity—lots of it or lack thereof—does not seem to be a factor. As previous studies have shown, vulvar pain patients are not likely to report childhood or adult sexual abuse. Also, the probability of sexually transmitted diseases is no greater in the vulvar pain population than the overall female population. But human papilloma virus does seem to be diagnosed more often in vulvar pain patients. (That could simply be because vulvar pain patients get tested for this STD more often; since HPV sometimes has no symptoms, many women may have it and not know it.) The high instance of HPV is also interesting because it supports the idea that the treatments for HPV, such as laser surgery, topical podophyllin, trichloracetic acid (TCA), and efudex (a topical chemotherapy drug applied to HPV warts), may contribute to the onset of vulvar pain. (Note: Many researchers don't think HPV is present more often in vulvar pain patients than in other women.)

Her Medical History

- Most sufferers (64 percent) did not have headaches or neck pain.

- Most (86 percent) did not have oral problems.

- 64 percent reported recurrent or persistent vaginal yeast infections.

- 73 percent reported recurrent or persistent bacterial vaginosis.

- 65 percent reported recurrent or persistent urinary tract infections (UTIs).

- 81 percent reported wearing glasses or contact lenses.

- 80 percent reported ear problems, mostly dizziness/motion sickness.

- Nose and throat problems were frequently experienced; 75 percent of vulvar patients complained of congestion.

- 83 percent reported musculoskeletal pain, primarily back pain.

- 67 percent reported digestive problems, primarily diarrhea/constipation.

- 60 percent reported urinary urgency and frequency.

- 75 percent reported nocturia (getting up at night to urinate).

- Dermatological problems were common with 75 percent reporting dry skin, healing problems, and easy bruising.

- Neurological symptoms of numbness, faintness, or weakness were reported at the extremely high rate of 90 percent.

- Less than 5 percent reported psychiatric illnesses, such as major depression, bipolar disorder, and schizophrenia. This rate is lower than the number reflected in the general population, which may be partly because seriously ill psychiatric patients aren't well enough to be on the Internet.

- Most did report milder forms of depression (89 percent) along with feelings of anxiety and panic (76 percent).

- Many reported the following disorders: irritable bowel syndrome (69 percent), interstitial cystitis (56 percent), Hashimoto's disease (28 percent), fibromyalgia (30 percent), and autoimmune/inflammatory diseases (30 percent).

What it all means. Vulvar pain patients reported more frequent vaginal yeast and bacterial infections as well as UTIs compared to the population at large. It is unclear what the relationship is between these infections and vulvodynia, but here are a few possibilities:

1. Vulvodynia may be masking itself with yeast-like symptoms. That leads many patients to self-diagnose and self-treat their symptoms with over-the-counter preparations, which may work to exacerbate their underlying vulvodynia. Similarly, physicians will also sometimes prescribe medications without an examination of the patient based on symptom reports.

2. Persistent infections themselves may cause the onset of irritated vulvar tissue.

3. The irritating treatments such as topical antifungals may play a role in the onset of vulvodynia.

They did not experience more frequent head or neck pain or oral problems, but did experience more frequent nose/throat, respiratory, digestive, and urinary problems—which is an interesting finding. The vulva, along with the intestinal lining, bladder lining, and respiratory tract lining, consists of mucosal tissue. It's possible that all mucosal tissues are more sensitive—and more inflammation prone—in vulvar pain sufferers.

Vulvodynia sufferers reported more musculoskeletal disorders. Why? Postural misalignments affect the muscles of the pelvis, which can cause or contribute to pelvic pain syndromes like vulvodynia. Another possibility is that vulvar pain patients will often reduce or eliminate regular exercise due to their pain and are therefore more prone to musculoskeletal disorders. Yet another possibility is that chronic inflammatory disorders, which seem to occur frequently in vulvar pain sufferers, can also cause muscle aches and pains and conditions such as fibromyalgia.

Dermatologic conditions were prevalent. Many vulvar pain sufferers reported they have fair complexions and lifelong histories of skin sensitivity. Tissue integrity in general, including vulvar tissue, may be compromised in vulvar pain sufferers due to skin sensitivity.

Neurologic symptoms occurred more frequently in survey respondents than in the population at large. This may suggest underlying nervous system instability or reactivity in patients. In one well-known model of pain called chronic regional pain syndrome (previously known as reflex sympathetic dystrophy), longstanding pain of peripheral tissue origin sets off a process of chemical changes. Those chemical changes cause nerves to be irritable—causing tissues to sense more pain than usual. Eventually, sensing this pain becomes a habit for the central nervous system; even after the peripheral tissue irritation is resolved. Another possibility for the high instance of neurologic pain in sufferers is nerve dysfunction in the pelvis due to childbirth, trauma, or surgery. Nerve dysfunction due to nerve compression can also happen after chronic inflammation of tissue or when disk enlargement in the lower vertebrae puts pressure on the nerves.

Those responding to the survey reported a low rate of occurrence of significant psychiatric disease. The numbers clearly show that vulvodynia is "not in your head." But patients' frequent reports of depression and anxiety are likely to be consequences of their vulvar pain and the effects it has on their lives. There seems to be a great need for supportive emotional therapy in treating vulvodynia.

Irritable bowel syndrome, interstitial cystitis, Hashimoto's thyroiditis, fibromyalgia, and autoimmune/inflammatory diseases coexisted with vulvar pain at a much higher rate than found in the general population. This finding is consistent with several scientific studies.

Her Sex Life

Intercourse: Most patients (71 percent) had not had sex with vaginal penetration in the past six to twelve months, even though most (58 percent) used to initiate intercourse and reported a history of pain-free sexual intercourse for an average of seven years.

Intercourse pain: A minority of sufferers (21 percent) reported primary introital dyspareunia, meaning they had pain on intercourse from their first attempts. Many more women (79 percent) experienced later onset of dyspareunia and vulvar discomfort. Of those women, many had five years or more of pain-free sex (52 percent). Nearly half (48 percent) of sufferers reported less than five years of intercourse pain; and more than half (52 percent) reported having it for more than five years. Most with intercourse pain (70 percent) experienced it immediately upon penile contact or during penetration. Fewer women (30 percent) reported pain that begins with thrusting or after intercourse. Initial symptom onset was described as sudden for 67 percent and gradual for 34 percent. The vast majority (96 percent) of patients reported sexual pain restricted to the vaginal opening and just slightly inside.

Pain location: For most, the pain is localized in a specific spot or spots (58 percent). Of these the vast majority reported pain localized to the bottom of the vaginal opening (91 percent) and only 4 percent reported pain predominantly or exclusively on one side. Others (42 percent) reported generalized vulvar burning; 18 percent of those surveyed reported both specific spots of pain provoked by intercourse as well as unprovoked general burning pain exacerbated by intercourse.

Relieving intercourse pain: Most (80 percent) had tried vaginal lubricants, but 90 percent weren't seeing any reduction in pain. Nearly all of the women (85 percent to 95 percent) had sought intercourse pain relief by changing sexual positions, engaging in more foreplay, and avoiding condoms. But 92 percent hadn't improved from any of these actions.

Sexual desire: Most (62 percent) were experiencing sexual desire less than five times per month. The remaining 38 percent reported six or more episodes of sexual desire per month. On a scale of 0 (least) to 10 (most), 55 percent rated their sexual arousal at five or below; 45 percent rate their arousal at six or above; 73 percent of patients reported their arousal level as much lower than before their vulvar symptoms began.

Sex and their partners: The vast majority of the women (92 percent) have discussed their pain with their partner. In most cases (68 percent), their partners were just as interested or more interested in having sex with them as they always were. Despite vulvar pain, most women (73 percent) still rated their relationship as "happy."

Masturbation and orgasm: Many women (44 percent) weren't masturbating. Those who did (40 percent) masturbated one to five times per month. The remaining 16 percent masturbated more than five times per month. Of those who masturbated, many (50 percent) achieved orgasm more than 75 percent of the time.

Orgasm: Some women (21 percent) were getting manual stimulation from their partners but only half of those women experienced orgasm as a result. Only 22 percent were receiving oral stimulation from their partners and less than half of them were experiencing orgasm as a result.

Attitude about sex: Half reported negative feelings about sex.

Sexual dysfunction: A few women's partners (6 percent) were experiencing erectile dysfunction. Difficulties in ejaculation were occurring in 15 percent of sexual episodes.

What it all means. Overall, the sexual data indicates that vulvar pain patients suffer significant sexual dysfunction. Levels of desire are significantly lower than before the onset of vulvar pain. Frequency of all forms of sexual behavior, including oral and manual sex with a partner and masturbation, are low. Orgasms occur less frequently during all types of sexual stimulation. Interestingly, despite suffering significant sexual dysfunction, only half of sufferers reported negative attitudes toward sex. There is a wide range of sexual consequences to vulvar pain. Although they are in the minority, some women maintain significant levels of sexual desire, frequency, and pleasure. Research is needed to help us understand all the factors, both medical and psychological, that affect the sexual consequences of vulvar pain.

Relationship issues, including finances, recreation, showing affection, friends, correct conduct, philosophy of living, dealing with parents, conflict resolution, and outside interests, showed levels essentially the same as those found in the population at large (Meana et al. 1999). This is a very encouraging finding. Many sufferers generally express fear that they will not be able to create or maintain intimate relationships in their lives due to their vulvar pain condition. Our data strongly suggests that this is not true. The great majority of those responding to the survey reported being in long-term stable intimate relationships with a high degree of partner compatibility and a high degree of relationship satisfaction. (As you will see later, single women may have more difficulty establishing intimate relationships after diagnosis. Unfortunately, the survey sheds little light on this issue.)

Her Pain

- 81 percent reported vulvar pain onset between eighteen and twenty-nine years of age.

- 68 percent reported pain onset to be within a twenty-four-hour period.

- 68 percent reported that initial pain was severe—they rated it at a high level.

- While a number of women (36 percent) said there were no identifiable factors that caused the onset of vulvar pain, most thought they could identify an association with sexual intercourse (32 percent), vaginal infection (24 percent), surgery/accident (8 percent).

- 45 percent had pain for four years or less.

- 55 percent had pain for more than four years.

- 25 percent reported a consistent level of pain, 33 percent reported high variability in pain and the remaining 42 percent reported some variability in their discomfort.

- The most common sensation of pain was burning (87 percent). Other sensations included stinging (73 percent), stabbing (51 percent), itching (50 percent), aching (45 percent), and drawing or pulling (33 percent).

- Factors that aggravated ongoing vulvar pain were sexual activity (86 percent), direct pressure (70 percent) urination (46 percent), menstrual cycle (44 percent), bowel movements (26 percent), diet (22 percent), and orgasms (20 percent).

What it all means. In summary, most women reported rapid onsets of vulvar pain at early ages as a result of identifiable events of vulvar irritation or trauma (such as surgery or an injury). Most sufferers had experienced several years of vulvar pain as well. The pain varied greatly from woman to woman, but was most often described as burning, stabbing, stinging, or aching. Major factors that caused or worsened vulvar pain symptoms were sexual activity, direct pressure (as with prolonged sitting, bike riding, or tight clothing), urination, and the menstrual cycle (most often symptoms were reported as worse premenstrually).

Diagnosis

Most women (53 percent) consulted three or fewer doctors before receiving their diagnoses. Some sufferers (21 percent) had to see six or more. Within a year of experiencing their symptoms, 42 percent reported that they received the formal medical diagnosis of vulvodynia. Unfortunately, 26 percent had to wait more than four years before receiving this diagnosis.

These figures are both sobering and also somewhat encouraging. There are many horror stories of women who see vast numbers of doctors for several years without receiving a diagnosis. Clearly, unlike other well-documented medical disorders, vulvodynia is not usually diagnosed in just one visit by just one doctor. Another view of the data is more positive. Since 42 percent of those surveyed reported receiving their diagnosis within one year of symptom onset, it's clear that more medical professionals are becoming aware of and learning how to diagnose vulvar pain disorders.

Treatments

In the survey, patients rated the treatments they had tried. (Full descriptions of each treatment can be found in chapter 4.) Respondents reported whether they thought these therapies were good-to-excellent or fair-to-poor.

Treatment	Good to Excellent	Fair to Poor
Vestibulectomy (surgical removal of the vestibule)	53%	47%
Interferon injections	50%	50%
Biofeedback (pelvic muscle)	46%	54%
Antibiotics	44%	55%
Rx pain medication	43%	57%
Topical anesthetics (lidocaine)	39%	61%
Avoidance of irritants	35%	65%
Hormones	34%	66%
Tricyclics (Elavil)	34%	66%
Anticonvulsants (Neurontin)	32%	68%
Antihistamines	30%	70%
Chiropractic	28%	72%
Physical Therapy	28%	59%
OTC pain medication	26%	74%
Guaifenesin	22%	78%
SSRI (Zoloft)	21%	79%
Oxalate diet/citrate supplement	21%	79%
Nutritional supplements	19%	81%
Antifungals	17%	83%
Antivirals	15%	85%

Baking soda douche	15%	85%
Acupuncture	13%	87%

What it all means. These ratings are not all that encouraging, but the first thing to keep in mind is that this data comes from a selected population of women who are visiting the vulvodynia.com Web site and are therefore still seeking treatment for their disorder. Furthermore, we do not have data on how long women used any of these treatments. It is not at all uncommon for treatments to take several months before showing any benefit, and many patients discontinue treatment prematurely due to uncomfortable side effects or false expectations of rapid relief. Most women have to try many different treatments before they find one that works for them. It is not known why some treatments work in some patients and not others. Remember that although all of the conditions we are looking at are called vulvodynia, this is in fact a disorder of multiple causation; different factors and combinations of factors are responsible for the pain in each patient, and different treatments may work relatively better or worse in individual women.

(**Note:** The majority of respondents had vestibulitis, not dysesthetic vulvodynia. Vestibulectomy and interferon injections should be used only in vestibulitis patients.)

Treatment Ratings

With information from the previous chart, we've list the treatments from the most successful one to the least. Remember: This list is based on the opinions of women (most of whom are probably vestibulitis patients) who have tried them—and these women are still having some pain.

1. Vestibulectomy
2. Interferon injections
3. Biofeedback
4. Antibiotics
5. Prescription pain medication
6. Topical anesthetics

7. Avoidance of irritants

8/9. Tricyclics and Hormones (tied)

10/11. Physical therapy/Chiropractic (tied)

There are some surprises in this data. Historically, due to a poor understanding of vulvar pain disorders and a lack of effective noninvasive procedures, prescription pain medications, as well as invasive treatments such as interferon injections, laser surgery, and vestibulectomy, were used to treat vulvar pain patients. As awareness of vulvodynia increased and patient advocacy groups developed, surgeries, injections, and prescription pain medications were highly criticized for their interference with sufferers' lives. Doctors started using less invasive procedures, such as biofeedback and avoidance of irritants, but as with most backlashes, this one took us from one extreme to the other—now more invasive procedures that have been proven helpful are too often shunned. Thankfully, in recent years, doctors have achieved a better balance of treatment options. Today vulvar pain specialists tend to treat patients with the least invasive therapies first, moving on to more invasive techniques if necessary. Vestibulectomy is still a top-rated method to achieve relief for patients. (Of course, the recommended treatment should always be based on what is most appropriate for the specific symptoms reported by the patient and the medical findings during examination.)

Because patients did rate vestibulectomy so high on the treatment list, we are reminded that we should never let politics and prejudice outweigh scientific medical findings when seeking answers. More importantly, for many patients, no single treatment, or sequence of treatments, but rather a combination of several treatments, addressing multiple underlying causes simultaneously, works best. Clinically, we have found that the practice of simultaneous, multidisciplinary diagnosis and treatment produces superior results.

The appearance of antibiotics ranked as the fourth most effective treatment suggests that many respondents had bacterial infections, such as bacterial vaginosis or urinary tract infections, as significant components in their vulvar pain. Either they were incorrectly diagnosed (vulvodynia can act like these infections), or they had infections coexisting with vulvodynia.

Topical anesthetics and tricyclics and hormones were ranked seventh and ninth, respectively. It is somewhat surprising that both the tricyclics (such as Elavil) and hormones (such as vaginal estrogen cream) were so far down on the list. They are probably the most conservative and frequently prescribed medical treatments. Perhaps medical practitioners need to pay closer attention to their patients to find out if these treatments are—or aren't—really working. Patients and doctors should also be encouraged to persist in using these for a long enough time, and to achieve adequate doses before giving up.

Finally, it is surprising that avoidance of irritants (soaps, laundry detergent, dyes) appears so far down on the list. Experts universally recommend these self-help options, and patients practice them frequently. Dietary regimens and antifungals for vaginal yeast did not make the Top Ten treatments—another surprise since these are often courses of treatment.

What to Expect at Your First Visit

If you suspect you have vestibulitis or dysesthetic vulvodynia more strongly than ever, of course, the next step is to make a doctor's appointment and try to find out for sure. Do your homework before going to an office visit. You want to see a practitioner who is, in fact, well versed on the topic. If your current practitioner is not, keep calling around until you find someone who is. Most specialists are either gynecologists or dermatologists, but some primary care physicians and urogynecologists may also be quite knowledgeable. Take your records and be prepared to describe your symptoms.

Your Medical History

During an appointment with a vulvar pain specialist, you will be asked some questions. Understanding these questions and preparing detailed answers will help your doctor diagnose and treat you more successfully and efficiently.

Do you experience pain on vaginal penetration during intercourse or when you use tampons?

Doctors seek to identify historical medical factors related to your pain to facilitate the diagnosis. They may also ask questions about your sex life, so they can advise you.

If you say you have dyspareunia, your physician will want to know if you've always had it, from the first attempt at penetration and thereafter (primary), or whether it began later (secondary). Your doctor will want to know whether you feel pain every time, or whether the pain coincides with your menstrual cycle, or is random. If you have more than one partner, can you discern a difference? Could pain be related to penis size? At this point you have a comfortable opportunity to share the status of your sex life. Your doctor needs to know how profoundly it is affected, so he or she can determine the most suitable course of treatment for you. Your doctor should be aware of your greatest concerns, and respond accordingly, so you should discuss whether you are more concerned about sex or relief from everyday pain.

Patients tend to use pads and tampons equally. Some find one or the other more comfortable. Your doctor will want to know if tampon insertion is or always was painful (to determine primary or secondary pain). In addition, if you report that tampon insertion and/or removal are painful, your doctor will suspect you have vestibulitis. Also, the string can be irritating for some women. Irritation from pad use (which may be caused by the bacteria on drying blood or due to chemicals and deodorants in the pad) may suggest dysesthetic vulvodynia, although pads can exacerbate all forms of vulvodynia. The advice you are likely to get is to use minipads without deodorant (like Lightday Ovals) and change them frequently. If you are a tampon user, avoid super tampons and leaving them in too long. (You want to discourage bacterial and yeast overgrowth, as well as vaginal abrasions.) Don't use tampons on light flow days; they can dry out the vagina and cause discomfort.

Do you experience pain localized in the area around the vaginal opening (vestibule) with pressure from prolonged sitting, bicycle riding, or tight clothing?

This question establishes your degree of discomfort. If you can sit all day long without pain, your problem may be less severe and less functionally limiting. Doctors want to know the degree to which your problem impacts your everyday life. Their ultimate goal is to get you back to living—and doing whatever you want without pain. So if your problem does sound more severe, they are likely to choose more aggressive treatments.

Do you experience burning or rawness in the vulva without provocation much of the time?

While the previous question focused on point tenderness and vestibulitis, an answer of "yes" to this one may mean that you have dysesthetic vulvodynia. As you know, once point tenderness on provocation is ruled out, dysesthetic vulvodynia becomes the more likely diagnosis.

Do you experience vaginal dryness?

Vaginal dryness is associated with dysesthetic vulvodynia. Women with this type of vulvodynia tend to be older—in their thirties through their fifties. Their bodies may be experiencing various changes in hormone balance, a factor that may cause dryness. That said, hormone deficiency might not show up in blood tests because it is not yet profound. But even a slight decline in hormone levels will affect the vaginal area first, causing thinning of vaginal and vestibular tissue and also dryness. Atrophic vaginitis, or thinning of the vaginal tissues, often goes unnoticed by doctors until the changes are more extreme as see in postmenopausal (elderly) women. Specialists will be looking for this, though, as dryness is not unusual in women with dysesthetic vulvodynia. If you experience dryness, you may benefit from small doses of locally applied hormones in the form of creams or vaginal rings or tablets. If you are menopausal, oral therapy may be used, but this may take longer to help the vulvovaginal tissues, so local treatment may be used together at first to achieve quicker relief.

Do you experience vaginal discharge?

Often, but not always, a change in vaginal discharge is a sign of infection. Everyone has some discharge, and it varies during your cycle. If discharge is bothering you or unusual, try to describe it in detail to your doctor. If it's white and cottage-cheesy, you may have yeast. If it's yellow and fishy smelling, it could be bacterial vaginosis. Some women with more severe cases of atrophic vaginitis will notice a thin, yellow discharge. Clear discharge or a small amount of milky or slightly grainy discharge—enough to leave a small streak on panties—is usually normal. That said, appearance alone is not enough to make the diagnosis. At least half of patients think they have yeast, and it turns out that they have something else. Sometimes they have bacterial infections or healthy ovulatory mucus discharge. Occasionally, patients have herpes or HPV.

Do you experience frequent infections such as vaginal yeast/bacteria or urinary tract infections?

As you saw in the results of Glazer's study, 60 to 70 percent of sufferers say they do experience recurrent or persistent infections. Other studies also show there is a high correlation between the two. One of two things may be happening, and your doctor will be trying to figure out which one. First, either you really don't have these infections; instead you've had vulvodynia all along. Or second, your frequent infections are directly linked to your vulvodynia. It is believed that the reasons why you get frequent infections are also the reason your vulvodynia occurs. There could be an underlying misfire in your immune system or your body's chemistry (this phenomenon is not yet well understood).

Also, if you have been treated by other doctors for "yeast infections"—which you may or may not have had—a vulvar pain specialist may suspect that a reaction to those courses of treatment is related to your vulvodynia or made it worse.

Treatment of one infection can further change the proportions of various bacteria that live in the vagina. And sometimes it takes a while for things to get back to "normal." Plain old patience can be crucial. Eating one serving of yogurt with live acidophilus cultures per day can be helpful in restoring a healthy balance of bacteria to the vagina. (Although you can have too much of a good thing; i.e., an overgrowth of acidophilus bacteria can produce the same symptoms and the same visual appearance as a yeast infection. Also, some women use acidophilus supplements, but careful analysis of these products has shown that often these tablets don't contain the species that are on the label!)

Do your symptoms cycle with your menstrual periods?

By looking at whether your symptoms coexist with your menstrual periods, professionals can see if your pain is hormone-related. For example, if your pain flares up premenstrually, your hormones may be the culprits. Birth control pills can be prescribed or changed to adjust estrogen and progesterone levels. In severe cases, physicians may give patients medicine to suppress their periods altogether. In addition, estrogen increases at other times of the menstrual cycle can cause pain in some women. Again, birth control pills may be prescribed or adjusted to decrease discomfort.

Does stress worsen your symptoms?

Many patients say their symptoms get better when they're on vacation, calm and relaxed, and not under stress. Stressful situations cause changes in the body that lead to increased pain. When anxious or overworked, we tend to go into fight-or-flight modes, meaning that under the influence of adrenaline, peripheral blood flow is reduced, muscles tense up, body temperature is decreased, and nerves become hyper-sensitive to stimuli. Anything that was already uncomfortable will become worse due to the body's natural biological reactions. If someone complains of pain during stress, and is constantly under stress, anxiety management may be effective in reducing symptoms. In these cases, doctors can prescribe drugs to reduce emotional reactivity, which will therefore reduce pain. Other approaches may include relaxation exercises, meditation/guided imagery, and yoga.

Are your symptoms worse during or after urination?

Foods high in chemicals called oxalates have been suggested as a cause of vulvar discomfort (Solomons, Melmed, and Heitler 1991). Oxalates are crystalline substances released in urine and may irritate vulvar tissue. If certain foods seem to make some patients worse, doctors will advise women to avoid them. Doctors may also tell sufferers to rinse their vulvas with water after urinating to wash off oxalates or acids that can be irritating. Health care providers may also advise women to drink more water, which dilutes urine and makes it less irritating.

Have you seen several doctors who tell you that they can't find anything wrong with you?

Often, women who have no visible cause for their pain *do* have vulvodynia. In Glazer's study, 50 percent of sufferers say they were diagnosed with vulvodynia within a year. The rest of the women may have been searching for answers for years—all the while being told that nothing was wrong with them while they still felt pain. Those women need to be reassured that something *is* wrong, and they can be treated.

Do you experience any related symptoms such as irritable bowel, urinary urgency and frequency, chronic fatigue, muscle pains and sleep problems, inflammatory problems, respiratory problems, skin problems, autoimmune problems?

As is frequently the case, there is something about the underlying physiology in some women that may be a common causal factor in all the above problems and vulvodynia. If you do have any of the above problems, you may be more likely to have vulvar pain disorders. A positive answer to this question is simply a huge red flag that, yes, you probably are more at risk for vulvodynia.

Have you experienced a reduction in sexual desire, frequency, or pleasure?

This helps your doctor pick the best form of treatment for you. If you are abstinent, and want to have intercourse, sexual therapy work may be needed. If you are sexually active, other symptoms will need to be attended to first. Your answer to this question helps your physician determine your feelings and satisfaction with your sexuality—and helps him figure out how best to help you.

In the Stirrups: A Step-by-Step of Your Exam

Remember, the diagnosis of vulvodynia is known as a diagnosis of exclusion. That means your physician has to rule out other causes of your vulvar pain. Since there is no specific test for vulvodynia, your doctor will base his or her opinion on your medical history, ruling out other illnesses, and by looking for redness, swelling, or pain in your vulvar tissue.

All in all, the exam will be much like a standard visit to the gynecologist—with a bit more attention to your vulvar tissues. Just so you know—and aren't surprised—by the exam a vulvar specialist will do, here are details of what you're likely to encounter.

First, the doctor will do the regular breast examination, to make sure there are no tumors. This is done to be sure that no breast conditions are present that might make hormonal therapies unwise even if they might otherwise be helpful.

Next, you put your feet in the stirrups like you always do, but what may be different in a vulvar specialist's exam is the detailed inspection of your vulva. The doctor will examine the tissue for abnormalities including atrophy (thin tissue), lesions like bumps, blisters or slits in the skin, areas of thickening, and changes in coloration.

Your doctor will look for scaly areas that are found in certain chronic or recurrent infections (tinea, candida, papillomavirus, herpes simplex) or chronic skin conditions, such as psoriasis, seborrhea, lichen planus, lichen sclerosus, and lichen simplex chronicus. The symptoms of these conditions are similar and treatments for one may affect the other. If the doctor suspects any of the above, or if you test positive for any of these ailments, you will be treated for them. If the diagnosis is in question, your doctor may take a biopsy. Sometimes a colposcope, a magnifying instrument, is used to look for these problems if they have not progressed to the point where they are visible to the naked eye.

After inspecting the vulva, before proceeding with the internal (vaginal) exam, he or she will also do the Q-Tip test, which involves using a moistened cotton-tipped applicator to apply pressure all around the vestibule. Now, on occasion, instead of looking directly at your genitals the way most ob/gyns do, the specialist will be looking at your face. Why? Certainly, the doctor isn't doing this to make you uncomfortable, but instead is looking at your facial expressions to see when you wince. If the doctor pokes you with the Q-Tip, your face is bound to show when and where it hurts. Rest assured that the doctor is not trying to hurt you, but just trying to find the exact location of your vulvar pain. Some examiners may ask you to give them a number from one to five to let them know whether your pain is mild, moderate, or severe. This also helps them monitor your progress at subsequent visits.

Next, the doctor will do the vaginal examination that you're probably familiar with. This involves opening your vagina with the help of a speculum, to get a clear view of your cervix and to take a swab of your vaginal fluid from your vaginal canal. This fluid will later be checked under a microscope for obvious signs of yeast and bacteria and to check your vaginal flora.

The rest of the exam will probably be pretty much what you're used to. The doctor may feel for tenderness in your bladder and other pelvic organs to make sure there aren't other factors that contribute to your pain.

If the doctor found candida (a yeast overgrowth) in your vaginal tract, you are like many vulvodynia sufferers. Most survey respondents, 62 percent, reported persistent or frequent yeast infections. The challenge for your gynecologist is to differentiate between candida and vulvodynia (Stewart 2001a). To make diagnosis even more difficult, some patients have both!

So your doctor has to rule out yeast as the main cause of pain, and therefore needs to see you when your symptoms are at their worst, and when you haven't been on any antifungals (such as Monistat) for at least two weeks. If you have chronic candida, it can take six to eight weeks to complete treatment and improve symptoms. If you continue to have symptoms of vulvar pain and dyspareunia even after a medically supervised course of treatment (not just the over-the-counter creams), vulvodynia is likely. Remember, frequent yeast and vulvar disorders can coincide, but separating them is crucial to getting a proper diagnosis. (Even if you have been diagnosed with vulvodynia, if your symptoms are suddenly or significantly worse, you should be checked to see if a vaginal infection is contributing to your "attack.")

If you've had pelvic or vulvovaginal surgery, childbirth, injury to the back or hips, you may have nerve damage that is causing dysesthetic vulvodynia. Since nerve damage is a factor, the physician should also evaluate you for tumors, a herniated disc, severe arthritis, spinal stenosis, or arachnoiditis. X-rays or magnetic resonance imaging (MRI) may be useful. Other ailments that are closely associated and often coincide with dysesthetic vulvodynia are interstitial cystitis, fibromyalgia, and irritable bowel syndrome. If you have these ailments along with vulvar pain, you will need to have your care coordinated carefully to have the best chances for successful treatment.

Chapter 3

Why Vulvodynia
Strikes

While the study of vulvar pain may still be relatively new, the problem of vulvar pain has been around for ages—and was even documented in ancient times. The first records involving pain during intercourse can be found in the Egyptian papyrus and the Talmud (Foster et al. 1995). Fast forward to Dr. Alexander Skene's *Treatise on the Diseases of Women* (1889). He describes a disorder characterized by "excessive sensitivity" of the vulva that causes females to "cry out in pain" when examined and touched with the doctor's finger. Vulvar pain was not mentioned again until the 1920s when Dr. Anthony H. Kelly wrote about uncomfortable intercourse due to sensitive areas on the mucosa of the hymenal ring (Kelly 1928). Real research didn't begin again until the 1980s when Eduard Friedrich, M.D., published medical reports that gave a standardized description of the disorder and penned the term vulvar vestibulitis (1987). Thus, the modern study of vulvodynia began.

Many Theories

What causes this disorder? Many researchers have tried to come up with answers. A brief discussion of some of their theories follows. We believe that all of these theories, even the ones that have been disproven, have led to better findings over the years, as different angles have been explored. So understanding what was once thought about vulvodynia can provide better insight into the current state of the field.

Vulvar experts still have varying opinions on the origins of vulvar pain. But recent research is showing that some of the theories blend together. For example, inflammation and nerve pain theories may very well go hand in hand. The hope is that forthcoming medical studies, theories, and clinical practices will yield more definitive answers. Once the causes of vulvar pain are fully understood, we will have higher success rates with treatment.

It's also important to remember that there are probably multiple causes of vulvodynia. The problem could be much like headaches—different people get them for different reasons.

Genetic Explanation

After not finding suitable treatments for a large number of patients suffering from vulvodynia, researchers began to look for genetic causes (Witkin et al. 2000). They found that vestibulitis sufferers with one form of a certain protein involved in inflammatory reactions had a greater susceptibility to develop prolonged inflammatory responses in their vestibules. Interestingly, it was already known that women with this protein who also had irritable bowel and lupus erythematosus were more likely to have severe inflammatory responses. So this research was important for two reasons. First, it showed that some women may be genetically predisposed to have vestibulitis. Second, it strengthened the argument that inflammatory responses of mucosal tissue all over the body are related. Perhaps this inflammatory process is the main predisposing factor for vulvodynia.

Inflammation and Mast Cells

In general, women with vestibulitis do have chronic inflammation (Chaim et al. 1996). Biopsies show that they have a greater number of mast cells in the area. These inflammatory cells are reactive and release histamine, a chemical commonly associated with allergic responses. Women with vestibulitis also show an exaggerated immune response that might be the result of the process of past or current infections, such as yeast (Nyirjesy 2000). This process may trigger the inflammation and symptoms of vestibulitis.

Even more recently, another researcher found that vestibulitis patients have an excess number of mast cells in their affected areas (Bornstein 2001). In addition, he also found more nerve fibers in this region than in women who don't suffer from vestibulitis. He hypothesized that mast cells, producers of inflammation, cause the growth of nerve fibers. And more nerve fibers mean there are more cells signaling pain to the patient's brain. This leads to vulvar hyperalgesia, which simply means supersensitivity to painful stimulation. (A sufferer feels more pain than a normal person.) It could also be that increases in the number of nerves leads to an increased (inflammatory) response to stimuli.

Still another researcher believes that an underlying inflammatory process is a probable cause of vulvodynia. The tissue of patients with inflammation shows an increase in the number of special nerve cells that make serotonin and CXCR2, the shared interleukin-8 receptor (Foster and Hasday 1997).

Concentrations of interleukin, a chemical that mediates inflammation, are also increased in women with vulvodynia. Put in simpler terms, Foster was able to identify excess self-produced, proinflammatory chemicals in patients' vulvas that seem to cause vulvar pain sensitivity (Foster 2001). Hopefully, his finding will lead to more effective pain medications. Now that chemicals that cause inflammation are better understood, it should be easier to develop drugs to combat the abnormality. Anti-inflammatory drugs have not been very successful so far.

Interstitial Cystitis and Irritable Bowel Syndrome

Whatever dysfunction exists in the inflammatory processes of vulvar pain patients seems to occur in their mucosal tissues. More specifically, areas of the vestibule are made up of transitional epithelium similar to bladder tissue. This may explain why many patients who have vulvodynia also have disorders such as interstitial cystitis and irritable bowel. For some reason, patients with any of these problems seem to have an abnormal predisposition to inflammation and a more extreme physical response to inflammation in their tissues. It may not be a coincidence that 25 percent of interstitial cystitis patients also have vulvar pain. Many vulvar pain patients also have interstitial cystitis–like symptoms.

Fibromyalgia

This is another disorder that often occurs in vestibulitis and dysesthetic vulvodynia patients. Fibromyalgia sufferers tend to have constant muscle and joint pain all over their bodies along with high levels of fatigue. Dr. R. Paul St. Amand has said that all vulvar pain is a manifestation of fibromyalgia, and treats his patients with guaifenesin. His theory and treatments have not been proven or disproven and remain controversial (St. Amand 1999.)

Various Trigger Points

The nerves of the vulvar region send pain messages to the brain. It appears that the nerves "short circuit" and keep reinforcing the pain impulse in sufferers (Marinoff 1995). Some researchers now believe that all vulvodynia is mostly a nerve-mediated disorder. (Doctors Stanley Marinoff and Maria Turner began the now-common practice of using tricyclic antidepressants to block nerves from sending pain signals.)

To get a little more technical, here's how it works. The vulva has nervous communication through three major nerves: the pudendal, ilioinguinal, and genitofemerol. The pudendal nerve originates from the lowest region of the spinal cord and has three branches: the inferior hemorrhoidal (rectal) nerve, the perineal nerve, and the dorsal nerve of the clitoris. This pudendal nerve transmits sensory signals from the genitalia and perineum along with supplying motor function to the pelvic floor and external sphincters of the urethra and rectum. The ilioinguinal and genitofemoral nerves originate higher in the spinal cord, in the lumbar region—they have sensory functions but no motor function. The ilioinguinal nerve transmits sensory signals from the inguinal, or groin, area, mons pubis, and anterior vulva. The genitofemoral nerve transmits sensory signals from the anterior vulva and the labia majora (Thomason 1999).

Many researchers believe nerve receptors transmit pain because of tissue injury. These nerve receptors are called *nociceptors* and pain caused by tissue and nerve damage is *nociceptive*. Nociceptive damage can be caused by a wide variety of factors. One is neurological compression, where the nerves are crammed together too closely. Other possibilities include stretch injuries, cutting of a nerve (during surgery or episiotomy), or viral infection of the nerves, such as herpes simplex or varicella zoster viruses. Nerve damage can also occur because of pelvic floor descent, which stretches the pudendal nerve. Again, nerve injury could also be caused by constant inflammation (possibly due to yeast or genetic predisposition, as previously discussed), which also damages tissue. Tumors, cysts, and vaginal surgery can harm the nerves, too. Other culprits are straddle injuries (from horseback riding, gymnastics, or bicycling), back, hip, and knee injuries, ruptured discs, and laser ablation of vulvar skin. Constant use of antifungals, steroids, or antiviral agents may cause tissue irritation and increase transmission of painful messages. And lastly, atrophy of the vagina due to a lack of estrogen may be responsible for tissue deterioration, with increased circulation leading to atrophy (also known as neuropathy.) Damage to nerves can lead to an increase in nerve endings as the nerve attempts regeneration.

One recent study in particular supports this vulvar pain theory: Dr. Nina Bohm-Starke found an increase in the number of nerve endings in the vestibule of vulvodynia patients as compared to other women (Bohm-Starke et al. 1998). Even more recently, Bohm-Starke showed that vulvodynia patients have much lower pain thresholds (that is, a greater response to pain) in their vestibules than other women (2001). Her research definitely shows that vulvodynia patients perceive more pain than other women.

Oxalates

Oxalates are natural by-products secreted in urine. In high concentration, they tend to form crystals. The typical shape of these crystals as seen under the microscope is similar to pieces of broken glass. Dr. Clive Solomons suggested that these crystals act as irritants that provoke vulvodynia (Solomons, Melmed, and Heitler 1991). In 1985, a woman who had severe vestibulitis that didn't respond to vestibulectomy or laser surgery went to Dr. Solomons who theorized that the burning sensations she was describing were similar to what you feel when you touch certain toxic plants, ones that are high in oxalates. He thought that high oxalate levels in the woman's urine could be causing the burning. A test of her urine did show she was excreting high levels of oxalate. To minimize those levels, Solomons put her on a diet that eliminated high oxalate foods such as spinach, strawberries, peanuts, and chocolate. He also prescribed calcium citrate to help inhibit oxalate formation. Within three months of trying this diet and the calcium supplements, the patient was better. In a year, she was completely symptom-free. Reportedly, the patient's symptoms recurred after she stopped the diet, but were resolved when she resumed it once again. Absence of those oxalates apparently stopped the burning.

And that's how the oxalate diet began. Many vulvar pain patients try it, with mixed success. Some doctors criticize the theory because it's based on one woman's success story—and have not supported the idea. For example, one doctor did a study measuring patients' and control groups' urine oxalate levels—they were exactly the same, suggesting that vestibulitis patients *don't* have increased levels of the substance (Baggish, Sze, and Johnson 1997). In another study, the oxalate levels of patients was higher, but only 14.3 percent of sufferers improved when they reduced oxalates from their diets and took calcium citrate supplements (Bazin et al. 1994). It's unclear, probably even improbable, that oxalates cause vulvodynia. But oxalates may irritate existing pain (Stewart 2001a).

Another negative for this diet: Many patients hate it and lose weight when they're not trying to do so (Witkin et al. 2000). Everything said, some women do see improvement and swear that it works for them. For more information on the low-oxalate diet, see chapter 5.

Yeast Infections

In the late 1980s, yeast was considered a common cause of vestibulitis. One group of researchers suggested that women who get many yeast infections develop hyperactive immune responses (Ashman and Ott 1989). They thought this happened because the antigens (identifying proteins) on the yeast organisms were similar to the patients' own antigens. As the sufferer fought off yeast, her body was also attacking her own antigens, and, even after the yeast infection cleared up, her body would keep responding to its antigens. Then she'd wind up with constant inflammation and irritation. It is true that some people have much greater response to even small amounts of yeast—or even to gentle touch.

In the early 1990s, seventy-one vestibulitis patients were compared to a control group of women who didn't have vulvar pain (Mann et al. 1992). According to this study, 80 percent of those with vestibulitis experienced multiple episodes of yeast infections. Only 20 percent of the control group had recurrent yeast problems. Interestingly, this study also found a significant percentage of allergic reactions in the same vestibulitis patients. That fact led the researcher to conclude that females with the disorder may be genetically more susceptible to vulvar problems. Mann hypothesized that once the cycle of yeast infections began, patients' autoimmune systems may have overresponded, causing inflammation and pain, and the irritation causes vestibulitis to develop.

A few years later, however, another doctor found that yeast was no more prevalent in women with the problem than in women without it (Bazin et al. 1994).

But whether pain is caused by oxalates, yeast, or the touch of a finger or tampon, the fact that women with vulvodynia have exaggerated responses to the same stimuli remains consistent.

HPV

Human papilloma virus (HPV) was also once considered a probable cause of vestibulitis. In one early study, 100 percent of vestibulitis patients tested positive for HPV (Turner and Marinoff 1988). Recent studies have disproved the notion that HPV is the cause of vestibulitis (Dennerstein et al. 1994), although several researchers still argue that HPV and vestibulitis are closely associated. Because a large portion of the female population has HPV, it's possible that vestibulitis patients were just tested for it more often than everyone else, leading doctors to incorrectly assume that HPV was the source of the problem. Most patients with HPV don't have pain (though mild itching or irritation can occur). It is possible that in women predisposed to vulvodynia, a greater irritation is felt.

Most patients with vulvodynia don't have HPV. It's possible that women with more severe cases of vestibulitis have increased sensitivity in their vulvar tissue due to HPV, or that the immune system's attempt to fight this virus results in inflammation, which makes the tissues more sensitive.

Again, the treatments vestibulitis patients have undertaken to treat HPV can certainly make vulvar pain much worse (Marinoff and Turner 1991). HPV is generally treated with techniques that destroy or remove the infected layer of skin, including applications of more or less irritating chemicals and drugs, freezing, burning/cauterization, and laser destruction. The pain experienced during healing leads to ongoing dysfunction in some women.

Why the Burning Sensation Occurs

The vulva has many sensory nerves. Researcher Richard Reid first introduced nerve sensitization as a cause for chronic vulvar irritation (Reid et al. 1995), because the burning sensation involves nerves, nerve mediators, and pain perception. When pain receptors, known as nociceptors, are activated, it is usually due to tissue damage. If the receptors are undamaged and working properly, they send pain and touch sensations along the C fibers, which are peripheral nerve fibers. But inflamed (damaged) tissue activates the nociceptors for prolonged periods of time, causing the nerve fibers to fire off constantly. Prolonged firing of the C fibers sensitizes the nerve cells in a part of the spinal cord called the dorsal horn. From that place in the spinal cord, neurons transmit pain to the brain stem and the thalamus, causing the sufferer to feel it. So the theory is that sensitized peripheral nerves cause the brain to begin perceiving normal touches and sensations the same way it perceives pain. In short, each stimulation is painful.

Psychiatric Disorders

As mentioned previously, Howard Glazer's recent survey showed that vulvodynia sufferers don't have any more psychiatric disorders than the female population as a whole.

Muscle Dysfunction

In 1987, coauthor Gae Rodke treated a young woman for pelvic pain and vulvodynia who happened to be a physical therapy student. Even after full therapy for her pelvic infections, she had persistent pain which, upon exam, was associated with spasms of her pelvic floor muscles. Rodke and her patient decided to try physical therapy, including biofeedback, to relieve the spasm. As the pelvic floor improved, her pain decreased—eventually resolving entirely. Over the next few years, several other women were similarly helped.

In 1988, Rodke began working with Dr. Alex Young, a professor of dermatology at Columbia University and director of the Cutaneous Vulvar Service of St. Luke's/Roosevelt Hospital Center. In 1991, they approached Howard Glazer, who is a pelvic floor muscle biofeedback specialist. They wanted to integrate muscle rehabilitation and biofeedback into their treatment regimen for patients who failed to respond to the usual medical treatments.

Biofeedback is an electronically assisted measurement of physiological processes, such as heart rate, blood flow, and muscle contraction. Through the use of highly specialized computers, a specific physiological process is translated into an auditory or visual signal so that the patient can learn to control it—and return that physiological process to more normal, stable, healthy levels.

Initially, Glazer was skeptical. He didn't believe that biofeedback, which teaches patients how to control their muscle responses, would be useful in treating these conditions. He thought any muscle abnormality in this area was probably the body's way of naturally "guarding" the person from pain—and probably did not have anything to do with the *cause* of the pain. It is well-known that in any area of the body where there is soft tissue pain, the local muscles become tense. He was not convinced that muscles were the cause of the pain; he feared that rehabilitating them would do no good because the primary cause of vulvodynia would just perpetuate the muscle instability and tension.

At the time, though, other treatments were limited to pharmacological and surgical interventions that had limited benefits, potentially disruptive side effects, and other risks. They were not ideal. So at the insistence of the vulvar clinic doctors, Glazer decided to try his biofeedback techniques.

He started by treating fifty patients with different types of vulvodynia. After several months of biofeedback therapy, he noticed improvement. The strengthening, relaxation, and stabilization of the pelvic floor muscles in many of these sufferers resulted in relief. Glazer was surprised. In 1993, Dr. Rodke reported these results at the congress of the International Society for the Study of Vulvovaginal Disease. Slightly more than 50 percent of the women who tried biofeedback therapy were completely free of pain at the end of treatment. And overall self-reports of pain reduction in the entire population treated were reported to be 83 percent (Glazer, Rodke, et al. 1995). He continued to follow the progress of "cured" patients—after three or more years, they were still free of pain (Glazer 2000).

Why Biofeedback Works

Originally, it was believed that muscle activity was a secondary process intended to protect the vulvar area from pain. The observation that decreasing pelvic floor muscle instability leads to pain relief, however, suggested that muscle instability plays an important part in creating, or at least maintaining, the pain.

Glazer and Rodke hypothesized that instability of the pelvic floor muscle maintains the pain of vulvodynia. A hyperactive and unstable pelvic floor muscle might cause a reflex or signal from the nerves of the pelvic floor to the nerves of the local spinal cord. Their initial study (Glazer, Rodke, et al. 1995) also showed that muscle stability was the only characteristic that predicted pain relief. Data from other studies (White, Jantos, and Glazer 1997; Glazer et al. 1998) supported the original findings that pelvic floor muscle instability is the characteristic that most differentiates vulvar pain sufferers from "normal" women. Those results indicated that stabilization of the pelvic floor muscle was a key factor in alleviating pain.

Whether muscle instability causes vulvar pain or whether it just perpetuates the pain from other sources of irritation is still unclear. Researchers aren't sure that pelvic muscle dysfunction is the original cause of discomfort. Nonetheless, several studies have shown that stabilizing the muscles will reduce pain—which is what really matters. Pain causes muscles around the soreness to clamp down, which immobilizes the area. As the muscle spasm carries on, it can alter the flow of blood to the area. This reduces blood to the local tissue, limiting the tissue's access to nutrition, oxygen, hormones, and auto-immune chemistry, all of which are necessary to heal irritated tissue. In addition, chronic pelvic floor muscle tension and instability causes further vulvar tissue irritation by releasing additional irritating substances such as lactic acid. Lactic acid aggravates tissue and muscle even more, creating pain and further muscle spasm. Another chemical, substance P, is also released from chronically hypertonic muscles. This substance specifically triggers pain-sensing nerve fibers, called nociceptive C fibers. You can thus see how dysfunctional pelvic floor muscles add to the vicious cycle of pain.

This type of phenomenon, previously known as reflex sympathetic dystrophy, is now referred to as chronic regional pain syndrome. To summarize, in this model of pain, there is an original trauma or irritation to the tissue, but the normal self-healing process is disrupted. The one key element in this process is the excess tension and instability in the local muscle, in this case, the pelvic floor muscle.

As with other possible causes of vulvar pain, we do not yet know why most "normal" women's vulvas automatically correct irritation. We do know that vulvodynia patients experience a self-perpetuating irritation.

How Biofeedback Eases Pain

The particular type of biofeedback used to treat vulvar pain is surface electromyographic (sEMG) assisted pelvic floor muscle rehabilitation. In the treatment of vulvovaginal pain, it is very specific and involves the use of highly technical instruments, computer software, home training devices, daily exercise protocols, muscle monitoring, and subsequent electromyographic evaluations. These evaluations work like an electrocardiogram, which records the heart muscle's electrical activity. Those lines that computers draw to signal each beat are done through electromyography. Pelvic floor muscle activity can be recorded the same way. The vulvar pain patient inserts a tampon-like device into her vagina, which senses the electrical activity of the pubococcygeus muscle, one of the muscles of the pelvic floor. Specific computerized equipment and software records the muscle activity and conducts a highly sophisticated statistical analysis of the electrical "signature" of the muscle, looking at events that can happen in as little as one-thousandth of a second. A specific series of measurements are made, such as the total amount of electrical activity at rest and during voluntary contractions. These, along with the speed of a contraction onset and release, the variability of the muscle during rest and contract periods, and the speed at which the muscle fiber is firing, are used to help pinpoint the exact nature of any pelvic floor muscle dysfunction.

Identifying specific abnormalities helps professionals like Glazer determine the appropriate ways vulvar pain sufferers can conduct home-based exercises to normalize their muscles. Patients are instructed to do a certain number of pelvic floor muscle contract/relax repetitions for specific periods of time. These exercises isolate the correct muscles and give the woman a sense of what those muscles feel like. She learns how to keep training her muscles at home using an intravaginal sensor and surface electromyographic biofeedback home trainer. These tools help her monitor her progress. All of the above therapy helps her stabilize her pelvic muscles without the use of drugs or invasive surgical procedures. (It's important to note that the patients' main focus is not to strengthen their pelvic floors in Glazer's protocol of biofeedback. Strengthening muscles that are already malfunctioning may make the pain worse by increasing the resting tension and instability in a muscle already experiencing excessive tension and instability. Instead, the patient will learn to stabilize those muscles by following specific exercises individually prescribed to overcome the particular muscle disorder found during the office evaluation.) Some patients do feel temporarily worse as they begin treatment even if they do everything right. With persistence, this effect is temporary.

The History of Biofeedback

Biofeedback has its origins in the late 1960s in the laboratories of Neal E. Miller, Ph.D., a psychologist at Yale and Rockefeller universities. Miller used biofeedback to demonstrate the capacity of animals and humans to self-regulate certain physiologic process which they didn't think they had control over—such as heart rate and blood flow. He hypothesized that voluntary control over these processes offered largely non-invasive treatment options for many serious disorders. He found that humans could learn to exert direct control over vascular constriction (narrowing of the blood vessels) to reduce or eliminate migraine headaches. The ultimate success of biofeedback means it is now used to treat all sorts of ailments, such as irritable bowel syndrome, heart disease, and chronic pain.

In the application of biofeedback to pelvic floor muscles, it was first used to treat incontinence (the inability to control bladder functions) after vaginal deliveries, and was first described for this application by Dr. Arnold Kegel (1948). Yes, this is the same Kegel of the well-known Kegel exercises for your pelvic floor muscles. Kegel was the first to point out that patients must receive feedback on the activity of the pubococcygeus muscle in order to effectively exercise this muscle. He invented the first device to monitor this muscle, the perineometer. Dr. Kegel's device was an intravaginal balloon called a manometer, which measured and gave patients feedback on the activity of their pelvic floor muscles. It was not until many years later that John Perry, Ph.D., first applied the newly emerging technology of surface electromyography to the pelvic floor muscle in the treatment of urinary incontinence (Perry and Whipple 1980).

Not All Biofeedback Is the Same

Glazer's protocol is the only method of pelvic floor muscle surface electromographic biofeedback that has proven positive results in the treatment of vulvovaginal pain disorders (Haefner and Kaufman 1998), and has met the scientific and medical standards to be published in several peer-reviewed medical journal articles. Other practitioners may claim to do pelvic floor muscle work or even biofeedback, but most are not conducting treatment in line with the proven parameters. Even if providers are conducting pelvic floor muscle surface electromyographic biofeedback, they are often using older equipment and protocols, developed for the treatment of urinary disorders, which are not as effective in the treatment of vulvar pain and may actually make things worse. It's important to find a specialist who is using the correct protocols and equipment and has received training in the Glazer protocol (check www.vulvodynia.com for a provider nearest to your area). If you are using another type of biofeedback or physical therapy, be aware that it has not been proven effective by scientific medical standards. You may be spending precious time and money on less effective therapy.

How to Find a Reputable Biofeedback Practitioner

Listed below are some questions to ask a potential therapist when you're looking for biofeedback therapy. You should not hesitate to ask your therapist these questions, and if you are not satisfied with the answers, try someone else. These questions, developed by Howard I. Glazer, Ph.D., and John Perry, Ph.D., were designed to help you evaluate a practitioner's level of competence.

"Will you personally be doing the biofeedback training, or do you have a technician, nurse, or aide who does the actual work?"

Biofeedback is labor intensive, so many physicians don't do biofeedback training with patients. A well-trained technician, nurse, or aide may be able to give you more time and attention helping you perfect your exercises and techniques.

"How many times have you treated patients like me?"

It is okay to work with a beginning practitioner; everyone has to start somewhere. Just make sure he or she is properly supervised and has been trained by someone reputable.

"What specialized training did you receive to do this work?"

Therapists who do biofeedback may be psychologists, nurses, or physical therapists. To be certified, they are required to attend several two- to five-day seminars every year on how to do pelvic muscle rehabilitation with biofeedback. You should see someone who's had at least one such workshop. Make sure that the workshop focused on chronic vulvovaginal pain syndromes, not just urinary or bowel symptoms.

"Are you a member of a specialized medical society or group, such as the International Society for the Study of Vulvovaginal Diseases (ISSVD)?"

Ideally, the practitioner should be a member of this or another reputable group focusing on vulvovaginal disorders.

"What is the typical outcome for your patients using EMG biofeedback for vulvodynia?"

In outpatient clinics, where most patients are in otherwise good-to-excellent health, there should be a cure rate of around 50 percent and an overall symptom reduction rate of around 85 percent.

"What is the expected outcome in my case?"

Symptoms are extremely variable and satisfactory outcomes will be different for different patients. You will have to think about your own physical condition in deciding what you consider a good answer.

"How long do you estimate the treatment will take?"

In general, nine months of diligent daily practice should get most otherwise healthy patients positive results. If your therapist doesn't have this skill, you might want to shop around. (By the way, it is considered good practice to keep training muscles even after you're pain-free—to prevent relapses.)

"How often will I get to use an EMG biofeedback instrument in my training?"

The more often you're able to do the exercises (hopefully twice a day) the better your chance for success. The best way to do this is to rent your own equipment (you can purchase it at the end of the lease if you like). Some practitioners will let you practice in the office or clinic under supervision, which may be helpful at first, but limits your access (and rate of improvement).

"Do you have vulvodynia treatment software running on a specialized biofeedback computer?"

The use of general-purpose, relaxation-type biofeedback software is not acceptable. There are several major companies that have developed software specific to evaluating and exercising the rather unique pelvic muscles. These programs also produce printed reports of your muscle condition to document your progress to the insurance company.

"Do you use special insertable vaginal EMG sensors, or just surface 'patch' electrodes?"

All of the major vulvodynia systems are designed to use insertable sensors, because they all give much more valid and reliable indications of pelvic muscle activity than external surface electrodes. Longitudinal electrodes have been shown to give measurements very similar to those obtained with inserted needle electrodes but without the risks or pain.

Chapter 4

Getting the Help You Need

Since most doctors aren't familiar with vulvodynia, it may be a challenge finding the right one to treat your condition. Many women see up to five doctors before they are even diagnosed correctly. And even if a physician can properly diagnose the problem, he or she may not know what to do with you next. Your goal as a patient should be to find a professional who is well-versed on recent vulvar pain research and therapeutic options.

Your best bet is to find integrative treatment. If there is a vulvar pain clinic in your area, you are bound to find people who know that the skin, nerves, muscle, and urinary and digestive problems and infections can all contribute to this problem and need to be treated together. There are two problems, though, for the average sufferer living in the United States and Canada. One, very few of these facilities exist. Two, even if you do find one, it may not be on your insurance plan, or it may not be affordable. The Internet can help you find the nation's vulvar clinics. (See appendix B.) Also, many teaching hospitals have collaborative clinics between dermatology and gynecology. If there is a major teaching hospital near you, contact the department of obstetrics and gynecology to inquire.

What about money? If your insurance won't cover or reimburse you, you have to decide whether you can make this investment in your health, which could, depending on your case, reach a few thousand dollars. You may first want to try doctors who are covered under your plan. You can also try to find a sympathetic doctor in your plan to work with you to try to get the insurance company to pay "out of network," so you can see doctors outside your plan. If you know you can't afford a vulvar pain clinic or if there just isn't one to be found in your area, you have to do what most women do: Work with the doctors you've got.

If that's your situation, begin by calling all of the gynecologists in your area who are on your insurance's list of providers. Ask to speak to the head nurse or someone who knows the office's level of interest and knowledge in vulvar pain disorders. Find out if the doctor sees patients who have vulvar pain. Avoid asking if the doctor knows how to diagnose and treat vestibulitis and dysesthetic vulvodynia because such direct questions may put the nurse on the defensive. Instead, ask, "Do you often see patients with vulvar pain? Are you able to help some or most of them?" If the nurse has no clue what you're talking about, this may not be the office for you. But often, even unknowledgeable nurses and doctors can point you to a doctor who *does* deal with vulvar pain. Now, on the other hand, the nurse may know what you're talking about, but not have solid answers. That's okay. Of course, the more detailed the answer, the better off you are. But if you find someone who knows what you're asking, you may be in luck. It may be worth an office visit.

You might also decide to go for consultation with an expert to get a diagnosis and plan for therapy and take this information back to your local gynecologist. All doctors are not created equal. And even the most well-known doctors may not be equipped to help you solve your particular problems. Whether you're paying for it or your insurance foots the bill, you want to make sure your doctor is treating you properly and with the respect your condition deserves.

That said, if you live in Leota, Indiana, or Eufala, Oklahoma, you might not find a professional who knows about vulvodynia. So here's what you do: As nicely and diplomatically as possible, find out if the doctor in question is willing to become familiar with vulvodynia. While on the phone, tell the nurse that you are willing to bring in medical journal articles on vulvodynia. You will supply the doctor with research and tell him or her about resources, such as the National Vulvodynia Association. You might ask: "Will the doctor be willing to work with me?" At this point, you may need to explain your situation. Maybe you've seen more than three doctors who told you your situation was "in your head," and meanwhile you have read about all of these women who were treated and got better. You have to explain that all you are looking for is help. By doing this in a non-accusatory, professional fashion, you are more likely to find a caring doctor who will take on your cause.

Develop a Great Relationship

Once you've found a knowledgeable or just plain sympathetic doctor or nurse practitioner, you have to keep your cool. Even though chronic vulvar pain can cause enormous emotional distress, it is important to remain calm and collected when you visit the office. Many women admit to being angry with the medical profession as a whole for ignoring their plight for so long. If you are angry, it's important not to take your anger out on your doctor. Other women are just overwrought with frustration. They may come into the office crying and bursting with emotion only because they're so desperate to find answers and make the pain go away. That reaction won't do any good either. If you are too upset or emotional, a doctor may not be able to understand you. Valuable information could be lost in the tears. Second, some doctors may prematurely dismiss angry or weepy patients as psychologically unstable. While this is an unfair assumption for physicians to make, it is important for you to avoid this label if you want to be taken seriously.

Instead of focusing on how the pain is ruining your life, it's much more useful for the doctor if you can describe your discomfort in detail. Before the visit, gather all of your medical records that pertain to vulvar pain. Maybe you saw a urologist years ago and a gynecologist in college. If you can get those records, or even jot down the treatments they gave you, that information will be helpful to your latest doctor. Write down the chronological development of your problem. When did it start? When did it get worse? What was done about it and when? List specific symptoms you have and write down when they occur. If you can, jot down all of the medications you've taken, whether they helped or didn't help, and make note of any side effects. Last but not least, write down a list of questions you want to ask the doctor.

When it's time for treatment, always make sure you understand the doctor's instructions. Ask questions in the office if at all possible while your case is on your doctor's mind, or call the nurse later if you need to clarify details. Discuss the options. Find out why the doctor chose a particular treatment. If you're completely uncomfortable with a procedure, let your doctor know. You may be wary of someone who suggests you try surgery or interferon shots first or says these are your only options. For some patients, though, surgery is the best option. In that case, you should be told exactly why such an aggressive measure is necessary for you. There are almost always choices of what to try first, so share your concerns while remaining positive and hopeful. Doctors find it harder to help those patients who are extremely negative or who refuse every treatment right off the bat. Keep things friendly and professional at all times. Try not to be frustrated or irritated—especially if this doctor is trying to help you. Instead, be informed and concerned. If after you get home, you have a significant question about the treatment, find out if you can fax a note to the doctor. Writing a note will insure that your doctor has the information he or she needs to properly answer your question. You're more likely to get answers you need.

Because many doctors are just plain overworked and overbooked, and because these cases are more time-consuming, they can't always handle all of their patients and appointments as quickly as they'd like. Keep this in mind if you find yourself struggling to get your doctor on the phone. The next time you see your doctor, ask for the best time and way for you to contact him or her. Always be courteous to the nurses and office managers since they're the ones who relay your message. Be as detailed as you can with every question you have. If you think you have a problem, make an appointment. If you have been squeezed in between other appointments, try to be respectful of other patients' time, too. This may not be the best time for an in-depth discussion or non-urgent questions. Make sure the office staff members know you appreciate their effort in getting you in as soon as possible. It will make it easier if you need their help again.

Overall, the better your communication is with the doctor, the happier you will be with the outcome. Establishing a good relationship will ultimately give you a better sense of control over your course of treatment. You will be able to participate in decisions and carry out your doctor's recommendations with a sense of confidence. Plus, an attitude of hopeful optimism can go a long way in keeping your doctor invested in your care.

What Doctors May Suggest You Try First

Your doctor will tailor your course of treatment to your history and major symptoms. But here is what one gynecologist and coauthor of this book, Gae Rodke, tends to do with her first-time patients.

Dr. Rodke asks patients to complete an extensive questionnaire and patient history form and bring it to the first appointment. This allows the practitioner to review the information before beginning the initial interview, and makes certain that important details are considered, such as previous therapies and how they worked. After a careful vulvovaginal examination, vaginal fluid samples are collected and viewed microscopically to make sure there is no other vaginitis present. Laboratory tests for various conditions, such as yeast and STDs, are sent, as needed. The patient is treated for those conditions first. Next, if she is complaining of burning, a small dose of tricyclic antidepressants will usually be prescribed. On the other hand, if the patient has a history of yeast infections, or tends to suffer from allergies, or Dr. Rodke sees that the patient's skin is highly reactive (i.e., sensitive), she may prescribe an antihistamine (such as Vistaril) to stabilize the histamine packets in the white blood cells. This can help keep skin reactivity in the vulvar region at a minimum (working much the same way that antihistamines decrease redness and keep eyes from itching and watering for people with allergies). Some doctors advise wearing white cotton panties and avoiding dyed underwear, but Dr. Rodke says the most important thing is to avoid trapping moisture near the skin. Unless you are sensitive to dyes or fabrics, the type of fabric is less important than avoiding a style of underwear that causes friction (e.g., thong-style underwear) or fits too tightly. Changing undergarments when necessary during the day or going without underwear under loose clothing when possible (especially when lounging at home or sleeping overnight) may enhance comfort. The new "breathable mesh" panties are very good for many women.

Dr. Rodke may suggest applying cold compresses to the vulva several times a day, using either plain water or Aveeno colloidal oatmeal solution. The patient can mix two tablespoons of Aveeno with a quart of cold water and apply it to the affected area with a cotton ball (just leave the remainder in the refrigerator). This easy-to-do treatment can soothe everyday discomfort. (See chapter 5 for more self-help options.) Drinking more fluids may also help. So can rinsing your vulva off with water after urinating (but be careful because overwashing can cause irritation).

Dr. Rodke also asks her patients to decrease high oxalate foods in their diets. (See chapter 3 for more information on oxalates.) Dr. Rodke consults with coauthor, Dr. Glazer, for surface electromyographic (sEMG) evaluations in patients with vulvodynia or vestibulitis to determine whether pelvic floor muscle dysfunction may be playing a role in the vulvar pain. If so, she suggests biofeedback, a technique of retraining your pelvic floor muscles. Dr. Rodke usually tries the above methods before considering more aggressive therapies, such as injections or surgery.

A Few Words About Your Health Insurance

Getting an accurate diagnosis and good treatment for vulvodynia can be an expensive process. Usually, sufferers see several doctors before finding a suitable one, and then they spend hundreds or thousands of dollars in search of a treatment that eases their pain or "cures" their symptoms. Hopefully, their health insurance covers the endeavor. Usually, it does, just as it covers the costs of most illnesses. Problems arise mainly because vulvodynia is still an unknown, misunderstood disorder. The problem is partly that the time and resources necessary for the complete evaluation of this problem are not "justified" by any one diagnostic code. If the doctor checks off all the codes that describe your symptoms and findings to justify the level of service, it may trigger the insurance company to reject the claim as "unusual," and require further investigation. This delays payment. Also, since many treatments used are "new" or "off label" (that is, they are FDA-approved for use in other conditions, but not specifically for this one), the insurance company may reject a claim for payment on the basis of "unproven benefit" or "not medically necessary."

This doesn't mean the treatment isn't a good idea (or your best chance at feeling better), it just means they consider it to not be eligible for payment. Different policies have different benefits and rules.

So be informed about the care you receive. If your doctor plans a specific procedure, call your insurance company to see if it is covered. In some cases, the billing clerks in your doctor's office are the most helpful. They know what office services tend to be rejected by insurance companies. If you can get one of them on the phone, find out if there are any red flags in the services your health care provider tends to render. You may ask, "Have other patients had trouble with companies reimbursing them for treatments? Do you have any suggestions for me that will help me get covered?" If you need lab testing, find out whether the doctor can (or will) use the lab in your insurance plan. If so, find out whether the tests need to be approved by your in-network doctor or insurance company.

Michelle, a twenty-eight-year-old vestibulitis sufferer, dealt with an insurance company snafu that cost her five hundred dollars. It turns out that her gynecologist runs very expensive, precise tests for several strains of HPV. The high-tech lab her doctor used wasn't covered in her HMO insurance plan. If Michelle had only known which lab her insurance covered and had requested that whenever possible the doctor use the participating lab, she could've saved herself several headaches and lots of time arguing with her insurance agents on the phone. She did need to have the sensitive, expensive tests run. (It turns out she *was* positive for a less common and more serious type of HPV.) If she'd known about the expense, she could have made arrangements to pay the extra costs little by little, or even saved for them, before the doctor's office clerk got upset about a mounting unpaid bill. In the end, her doctor agreed to allow her to pay the bill over time. Remember, no matter what your insurance company may tell you, your doctor will hold you, not your insurance company, responsible for payment, if the doctor does not fully participate in your plan.

Sometimes, however, an insurance company may refuse to pay for a service that should be covered, such as specialized prescriptions or surgery. In this case, your physician's help in the matter is crucial. Usually, the doctor will need to write a letter to the insurer detailing the services and explaining the reasons they were necessary. If possible, give your physician a few relevant medical articles (or pages copied from this book) to attach to the letter. Again, since vulvodynia is often misunderstood, the insurance company may respond favorably to explanations and educational materials.

As you can see, it's important for you to be well-informed about your insurance company's rules. If you are staying with an in-plan provider, charges for the workup, office visits, and tests are set (they're prenegotiated by the doctor and insurance companies). If you go out of the plan, ask to be informed in advance—whenever possible—of extra tests and procedures and whether they can be done "in network." If you have another participating doctor who is cooperative—and knows you're trying to get outside help for vulvodynia with a group of non-participating specialists—he or she may be able to save you significant amounts of money by handling the tests and lab work.

Of course, finding a knowledgeable doctor who can both treat vulvodynia and participates in your plan is the greatest challenge. If it turns out that no knowledgeable physician in your area works with your insurance company, you'll have to consider paying the bill. (But keep in mind that getting better is your top priority. It might be worth your money to go to a specialist or vulvar clinic even if it's not on your plan. Think of it as an investment in your health.)

If you choose to work with a less informed physician, it is worth considering paying with your own funds for a one-time evaluation with a specialist. Consulting with an expert may help you assess whether you are receiving a correct diagnosis, and he or she can provide suggestions of what is best to explore with your local in-network doctor.

Your Treatment Options

For more in-depth information on the above methods of treatment—as well as several more—study the detailed descriptions that follow. We want to provide you with a reliable guide that will help you understand your medical options—why they're prescribed and how they work. A beginning knowledge of the usual treatments will also provide you with the knowledge you need to ask your medical care provider the most informed and helpful questions. The treatment options below are presented in alphabetical order, not according to effectiveness.

Acupuncture

According to a recent study, this ancient therapy benefits vulvar pain patients (Powell and Wojnarowska 1999). In the study, 75 percent of the women—all with longstanding vulvodynia that didn't respond to different treatments—improved greatly. A small percentage even claimed they were completely cured after ten weekly sessions. How is this possible? Researchers believe that the needles relieve pain because of their ability to dull pain fibers (called A delta fibers). It's possible that acupuncture treatments actually turn off these overactive, malfunctioning pain fibers. Since the sample size of the study was so small—only twelve women participated—more research on this treatment is needed.

If you decide to try acupuncture, do a thorough background check of the practitioner. Talk to previous or current clients if you can. (Interestingly, the acupuncturist doesn't need to know exactly where your pain is for you to experience benefits from this technique, although it's probably best to let the practitioner know why you're there.) Many women have reported deep relaxation and temporary pain relief after receiving acupuncture. Another reason acupuncture may work is that it is thought to cause the release of endogenous opiates, the body's natural painkillers, which interrupt the vicious cycle of pain.

Antibiotics

The use of antibiotics is highly controversial. Your doctor may want you to take them, especially if your white blood cell count is high or if your Bartholin's glands are especially inflamed. Many women have reported that antibiotics seem to help at first but then cause a "rebound" effect where the pain returns—only worse. Some sufferers believe that their vulvar pain actually began with the use of antibiotics. For this reason, many women are not eager to try more antibiotics.

There is no direct link between antibiotic use and vulvar pain, but antibiotics can definitely lead to yeast infections. Repeated courses of medications can lead to harmful bacteria resistant to antibiotics. Both are good reasons to question your doctor for pre-scribing antibiotics for your condition. (One exception is if your doctor has diagnosed you with persistent vaginal B-strep, which is treatable with penicillin.)

Anticonvulsants (or Anti-epileptics)

Commonly, these meds are used to prevent seizures. But for patients with vulvodynia, it is believed that central and peripheral pain nerve sensitization may be one of the underlying causes of the pain. The idea behind using anticonvulsants for vulvar discomfort is that they raise a person's level of pain tolerance. The drugs make nerves able to withstand more stimulation, so hopefully those nerves won't fire off pain signals as quickly or as often, and the patient won't feel as much discomfort. Women with dysesthetic vulvodynia (as opposed to vestibulitis) who report spontaneous "stabbing" or "shooting" pain seem to have the most success with this therapy.

Anticonvulsants are typically taken at higher doses than antide-pressants. (See more information on tricyclic antidepressants later in this chapter.) Because of their substantial effect on the central ner-vous system and the common side effects, anticonvulsants should be tried only if antidepressants fail to do the job, or if the side effects are persistent and unacceptable. Sometimes doctors will prescribe both medications together in an attempt to produce the best therapeu-tic response and least side effects.

The most widely used anticonvulsant is Neurontin (gabapentin, generically). Dosages can be anywhere from 900–4000 milligrams per day, usually divided into three equal dosages. Side effects, while much less problematic than with the older convulsants, may include sleepiness, ataxia (the inability to coordinate voluntary bodily move-ments, such as walking), fatigue, dizziness, the involuntary rapid movement of the eye, weight gain, and fluid retention.

Another anticonvulsant is Tegretol. It is usually given in dos-ages of 400–800 milligrams daily, with initial dosages starting at just 100 milligrams. Starting with lower dosages and slowly increasing them will reduce side effects such as dizziness, drowsiness, nausea, unsteadiness, and vomiting. You must see your doctor regularly when on this drug, so your blood can be properly monitored. A newer version, Trileptal, has milder side effects and does not require blood monitoring.

Remember it takes several weeks at higher doses (not the starter doses that get your body used to the medicine) to judge whether these drugs will work for you. So if you start them, expect a wait time, and try not to be discouraged if relief seems delayed. Most of the side effects of these drugs decrease with time, so allow yourself to get used to them.

Anti-inflammatories

Regardless of the underlying reasons *why* the vulvar skin becomes inflamed and causes vulvodynia, anti-inflammatories may be useful in attacking the inflammation and decreasing discomfort. While over-the-counter anti-inflammatory drugs such as ibuprofen (e.g., Motrin or Aleve) have not been very helpful, other newer drugs are more promising. Some experts think other anti-inflammatories may be of future use for vulvar pain. These include Celebrex and Vioxx, which are commonly used for arthritis. They selectively target and inhibit prostaglandins, hormone-like substances that may cause the inflammatory response. They may or may not work for vulvar pain as well. More study is necessary. Preliminary research on the generic drug prenosine for use in vulvodynia patients is also promising (Sand Peterson and Weismann 1996).

The good news: There are some home remedies you can try right now. These are some of the least invasive and cheapest ways to soothe vulvar pain. Some to try are zinc lotion (Anusol, non-steroid formula), A&D lotion (diaper rash product), Aveeno compresses, calendula ointment (homeopathic or an herbal salve), comfrey ointment, pau d'arco ointment, St. John's wort ointment (note: may have a different efficacy than oral St. John's wort), black teabags (not herbal) moistened with either warm or cold water (note: You can get a caffeine high from intervaginal absorption), vitamin E oil (from the caplet). Unpetroleum jelly, made from the castor bean, makes a nice barrier if urinary symptoms are an issue. It can be very soothing, but like all oil-based products, it can break down latex condoms—so if you use it, try polyurethane condoms instead.

See chapter 5 for more detailed information on these and other at-home treatments.

Anti-virals

Anti-virals, such as acyclovir (Zovirax), famcyclovir (Famvir), and valcyclovir (Valtrex), are helpful in patients who also have herpes simplex virus. Since herpes lives in the nerve roots, it can cause pain, as seen in patients with shingles—which is a delayed reactivation of the chicken pox virus, often from long ago. Patients with genital herpes can have pain associated with prodromes (the time before lesions occur) as well as with the lesions themselves. Taking these drugs to suppress recurrences can remove one more pain-causing factor from the mix. They are safe and have very few side effects

Anxiolytics

These are anxiety-reducing or sedative drugs. The older class of them, called the benzodiazepines like diazepam (Valium), work by increasing the amount of the neurotransmitter GABA in your brain. They may help reduce vulvar pain because they lessen sympathetic arousal. Put more simply, when your body goes into "fight/flight" mode, it senses pain more acutely. And pain can make you even more anxious, starting a self-perpetuating cycle. Anxiolytics work by calming the patient down. So it's not surprising that their side effects include mental sluggishness and drowsiness. Unfortunately, another major side effect of these drugs is that they can be addictive. Newer anxiolytics have been developed that target different neurotransmitters and are less addictive.

Biofeedback

Using biofeedback for vulvovaginal pain is a relatively new concept that the medical community is just starting to use (see chapter 3). Traditionally, biofeedback involves electronically assisted measurement of a biological event and providing information about these events to the patient using visual or auditory feedback. In vulvar pain patients, it is used to help teach them to control the electrical activity of their pelvic floor muscles. The idea behind biofeedback is to stabilize the resting electrical activity of the pelvic muscles. This treatment has proven to be extremely effective in reducing pain of vulvar patients. One study showed that 50 percent of vulvar pain patients reported total absence of symptoms and the average report of improvement in the entire population treated was 83 percent after sixteen weeks of treatments (Glazer, Rodke, et al. 1995).

Vulvar pain patients have been shown to have excessive and unstable levels of electrical activity in their pelvic floor muscles—a natural response to protect the area from pain. This book's coauthor Howard Glazer developed a protocol to help patients rehabilitate these muscles. He uses such instruments as a small intravaginal device to detect pelvic floor muscle electrical activity and a biofeedback instrument to deliver this information to the patient. Then he shows patients how to activate and release the muscles to reduce excess resting instability and hypertonicity. Relaxing the muscles works to reduce the release of local irritative chemistry and increase blood flow to the area, restoring it to the status of healthy, pain-free tissue. Dr. Glazer's patients, both vestibulitis and dysesthetic vulvodynia sufferers, typically see significant improvements in their symptoms after nine months of at-home therapy with intermittent follow-up office visits.

A major drawback of biofeedback is that it's hard to find a knowledgeable practitioner. Be aware of the differences between the regimen used in the Glazer protocol and other forms used by some physical therapists and urologists to treat other conditions. The studies showing the response rates quoted in this book all used the Glazer protocol. While other methods or protocols may turn out to be helpful, there are not yet good data for comparison. Another problem with biofeedback is that it can be expensive. But with some explanation, many insurance plans cover the therapy. Finally, biofeedback takes a good deal of persistence and discipline, as the average pelvic floor muscle exercise prescription for home training is twenty minutes, twice a day, for an average treatment period of nine months.

Estrogen Therapy

John Willems, M.D., at the Scripps Clinic in San Diego, advocates the use of estrogen cream (Estrace)—not to increase estrogen levels throughout the body but only in the vulvar vestibule. A centimeter or quarter-inch of estrogen cream applied to the vulvar vestibule each night may provide comfort to some sufferers. It helps thicken the top layers of skin at the opening of the vagina, which can insulate the nerve endings that send pain signals. It can also increase blood flow to the area. Due to the small amount used and limited absorption in this area, blood levels of estrogen do not increase using this method, and it is considered very safe, meaning it doesn't increase the patient's chances of getting breast or endometrial cancers. (Note: There has been a lot of controversy over hormone replacement therapy because sytemic estrogen replacement [with pills or patches] may or may not be associated with increased breast cancer risk. Re-estrogenizing the vagina using minimal doses as described here is not reported to increase cancer risk.)

Topical estrogen in larger doses (several times as much) is usually prescribed to post-menopausal women as a form of hormone replacement therapy. Women of all ages with vulvodynia may benefit from using it as well. Sometimes doctors not familiar with essential vulvar pain disorders are reluctant to prescribe it for younger women, however. Many women experience mild irritation with Estrace possibly due to an irritating ingredient in the cream. For women who find the commercially available creams irritating, a qualified compounding pharmacist can mix an equivalent percentage of estradiol in a preservative-free emollient base. Note: Such a pharmacist may be difficult to find so try the Women's International Pharmacy (see appendix B).

There is also an intravaginal estrogen tablet (Vagifem) and an insertable device called Estring that deliver estrogen to the vagina. Estring works by systematically releasing estrogen into the vagina. Unfortunately, the device can sometimes be uncomfortable for women who are prone to pelvic muscle spasms.

Estrogen therapies are inexpensive, unobtrusive, and somewhat successful. Though they do not provide a cure, they are helpful in managing vestibulitis (Stewart 2001b), especially when used in conjunction with other therapies like biofeedback and tricyclic antidepressants. A note of caution is that local vulvar or vaginal estrogen should not be used in the presence of an active yeast infection because estrogen supports the growth of yeast.

Immune System Modulators

In the 1980s, human papilloma virus (HPV) was considered a major cause of vestibulitis. While that notion is not as widely held today, many women with vestibulitis do have the presence of HPV in their vestibules. So interferon is still in use. Interferon is an agent that enhances the immune system, thereby enabling women to eliminate the virus and hopefully the vulvar inflammation also. It is administered via injection, either locally, by injecting it directly into the vestibule, or systemically, by injecting it into the arm or upper thigh muscle tissue. Administering the shot locally is preferred, due to a much lower recurrence of pain in the years following the treatment (Bornstein, Pascal, and Abramovici 1993).

To be a candidate for interferon injections patients must, of course, test positive for HPV. Some doctors may be interested in killing off wart viruses with heat, or by acid removal—both of which can irritate the vestibule even more. Others will try the interferon shots to try to rid the body of the virus. The downsides to the shots: They are expensive; it's uncomfortable to get shots in the vestibule; and shots must be administered nine to twelve times, usually three to four per week for a month. The upside is that 92.3 percent of patients will test negative for HPV eight weeks after the last injection (Ledger, Jeremias, and Witkin 2000). The success rate is reported to be 38.5 percent.

There are two types of interferon, alpha and beta. Beta was more recently synthesized in Israel, and has fewer side effects than alpha interferon (Bornstein, Pascal, and Abramovici 1993). But all in all, the type of interferon used has only a slight significance. In either case, the drug sometimes causes women to feel temporary flu-like symptoms, such as malaise, muscle aches, and low-grade fever. Benefits from interferon may not be apparent until months after the treatment is completed.

Low Oxalate Diet

As explained in chapter 3, this form of treatment was developed by Clive Solomons, Ph.D., a biomedical researcher. He believes that reducing the amount of irritating oxalates found in the urine helps to prevent vulvar burning (Solomons, Melmed, and Heitler 1991). When oxalates are high in concentration, they form crystals. Oxalate crystals, known to cause burning in the skin, resemble small pieces of broken glass when seen under a microscope. To minimize a vulvodynia sufferer's oxalate levels, foods with high oxalate content must be eliminated. These include broccoli, spinach, strawberries, peanuts, and chocolate (see the list that follows of low- and high-oxalate foods). Calcium citrate (such as Citracal), an over-the-counter product, also helps prevent oxalate formation. Women on the low-oxalate diet are often advised to take 500 milligrams of calcium citrate three times a day before meals. (As a beneficial side effect, calcium helps prevent osteoporosis.) If the calcium causes any constipation, a combination formula including magnesium can be helpful.

While there is still debate on the oxalate theory, this approach is non-invasive, inexpensive, and relatively easy. So it is often the first option doctors suggest to their patients.

Below is a short list showing the relative oxalate content of common foods. It is most important, obviously, to avoid those foods highest in oxalate content. Foods with moderate oxalate content may be okay with increased water intake. As you will see, a low-oxalate diet may be hard to follow because so many staples are off-limits. And remember, before going on any diet, you should consult your physician, especially if you're pregnant.

Note: Following this diet strictly can reduce urinary oxalates by about 20 percent. This may be enough to make a difference, but it is possible to further reduce the concentration of oxalates (and other urinary irritants) by 50 percent just by drinking twice as much water!

Oxalate Quantities in Foods

Highest Oxalates of Ten Milligrams or More (Avoid These!)

spinach
peanuts
~~celery~~
blueberries
~~strawberries~~
chocolate
~~baked beans~~
~~okra~~
summer squash
~~sweet potatoes~~
eggplant
wheat bran
tea

Moderate Oxalates of Two to Ten Milligrams

apples
oranges
peaches
pears
pineapples
carrots
corn
broccoli
tomatoes
asparagus
~~sardines~~
cranberry juice
coffee

Low Oxalates of Two Milligrams or Less

bananas
grapefruit
melons
avocados
cauliflower
mushrooms
green peas
onions
eggs
cheddar cheese
poultry
lemonade
milk

Tricyclic Antidepressants

As already emphasized, it's important not to confuse the more common use of these medications with their use in controlling vulvodynia. Although these medications are used primarily to lower anxiety and decrease depression, this does *not* mean your vulvodynia is "in your head." Nor is your vagina "depressed."

Instead, there are biological reasons that tricyclic antidepressants work for dysesthetic vulvodynia patients (Edwards and Wiojnarowska 1998). These drugs alter the transmission of pain impulses. How? They modify the levels of your natural chemical messengers, called neurotransmitters. Also, tricyclics change the transmission of the chemicals norepinephrine, acetylcholine, and serotonin between the nerve cells. The bottom line is that the brain simply doesn't receive the pain messages, and if all goes well, the vulva doesn't hurt.

Most commonly, doctors will prescribe amitriptyline (Elavil), desipramine (Desipramine), nortriptyline (Pamelor), doxepine (Doxepin), or a combination of perphenazine and amitriptyline (Triavil) to their vulvar pain patients. They are prescribed in lower dosages for vulvar pain than they are for treatment of depression. Doctors will usually start patients off with a very low dosage and slowly increase it to minimize side effects. It may take up to three months to get to the dosage that finally offers some relief; approximately 50 to 150 milligrams are usually needed but some vulvar pain patients report improvement with as little as 10 milligrams. If the patient does experience a reduction in pain while on this drug, the dosage will be decreased after a few more months so that the sufferer takes as little of the medication as possible. Tricyclics need to be taken with food to minimize upset stomach, and they should not be taken with certain other drugs. The medication increases the effect of alcohol and can cause drowsiness. It cannot be combined with Tagamet, Prozac, thyroid medications, or drugs that improve breathing, such as Ventolin. Patients with irregular heartbeat or palpitations should be cautious.

Side effects may include fatigue, rapid heartbeat, and hypotension (lowering of blood pressure). Dry mouth and constipation may also be experienced, as well as confusion, short-term memory problems, impaired concentration, nervousness, increased appetite, and sun sensitivity. These irritating effects tend to decrease

as the body adjusts to the medicine. Some can be easily
acted—for example, if you take this medicine, wear sunscre€
you feel drowsy, take the medication at night instead of in th⌐ ₘₒᵣₙ-
ing. If side effects persist or prove to be intolerable, different tricyclics can be substituted. Many women have the best luck with
desipramine; it seems to cause the fewest side effects (Foster and
Duguid 1998). If sufferers don't have any relief from this drug after
taking full dosages for three months, other types of treatments should
be tried.

Other Antidepressants

The New SSRIs

The selective serotonin reuptake inhibitors (SSRIs), such as
Prozac, Zoloft, and Paxil, used to treat obsessive-compulsive and
depressive disorders, do not have a significant medical literature
reporting their effectiveness in treating vulvodynia patients. They do
have fewer side effects than the older tricyclics, but they do not have
any demonstrated effect on the mechanisms of neuropathic pain. It is
likely that any benefit seen from these medications is due directly to
their antidepressant and anti-anxiety properties.

Trazodone Hydrochloride (Desyrel)

This non-tricyclic antidepressant differs slightly from other
antidepressants and may have fewer side effects. It does, however,
seem to have central nervous system effects such as confusion or
agitation.

Perphenazene (Trilafon)

In addition to functioning as an antidepressant, this medication
also works as an antihistamine and anticholinergic agent, which can
be especially useful for vestibulitis patients, as well as anyone with a
lot of sensitivity in her vulvar skin. Its side effects include drowsiness, blurred vision, and discolored urine.

Hypericum (St. John's Wort)

This herbal antidepressant has produced results comparable to SSRIs in clinical trials. But it seems to act more like a tricyclic. Since St. John's wort is available over-the-counter and unregulated by the FDA, the trick is finding a manufacturer who sells a quality-controlled product. The active ingredient in St. John's wort is hypericin. You should buy standardized extract containing 0.3 percent hypericin. The usual dose is 900 mg per day. It can take up to four weeks to see any improvement in vulvar discomfort. It goes without saying that it's always best to take this medication under the care of a physician—even though it's a nonprescription supplement. St. John's wort is a phytoestrogen that has potentially dangerous interactions with other herbs that affect hormonal balance, such as licorice root. It may make the birth control pill less effective for contraception. Caution: It's extremely important that you do not take an MAO-inhibitor, such as Nardil or Parnate, while taking St. John's wort. Another side effect is sun sensitivity. That said, some patients have reported improvement in vulvar pain using this herbal remedy (see survey results reported in chapter 2).

Vestibulectomy

Vestibulectomy is a surgical procedure that is only helpful to vestibulitis sufferers. (It is not useful in patients with generalized burning.) The idea is to remove afflicted tissue and replace it with less sensitive vaginal tissue. And it does seem to work. The particular surgery with the best success rate is modified vestibulectomy, which involves the removal of a horseshoe-shaped area of the vestibule. The posterior wall of the vagina which is quite elastic is freed up and is extended down to cover the area removed, and stitched without tension over the area where the excised vestibular tissue was located. This creates a cushion of thick, more elastic tissue around the vaginal opening and helps to make intercourse more comfortable. With women whose pain is localized point tenderness, confined exclusively to the vestibule, the success rate is 76 percent (Bornstein et al. 1997). Sexual therapy following the surgery increases the success of surgery and is strongly advised (Stewart 2001b). Dr. Rodke recommends the gentle use of a vaginal dilator starting about three weeks after surgery to gradually get patients ready for intercourse and to keep the scar line from becoming tight in the meantime.

Complications from the procedure are rare, but some women do deal with separation of the stitches, blood collections or clots under the surgical area, infection, uneven healing, or tender knots of scar tissue along the suture line. Occasionally a minor procedure may be necessary to correct these problems. Closure of the Bartholin's duct may rarely lead to cyst formation.

Another version of the surgery involves removing the most tender areas of the vestibule, as performed by Gordon Davis, M.D., at the University of Arizona College of Medicine. Again, high success rates have been found. Ten out of twelve women reported no pain after surgery, and the remaining two reported less discomfort (Goetsch 1996). This procedure is less invasive and can be done in the doctor's office using local anesthesia. Unfortunately, once the most painful areas have been removed, other problem areas may become more noticeable. Tender scarring can also occur with this procedure. Another drawback is that vaginal advancement is not part of this technique, so the scars are at the introitus, where they are more likely to cause discomfort during intercourse.

Although there have not been comparative studies reported in the medical literature, the complete modified vestibulectomy with vaginal advancement and perineoplasty is presently preferred by most specialists.

At one time, CO_2 laser vaporization of the vestibule was used to cure vulvar pain associated with HPV. Healing took too long and patients complained of scarring that led to thinner, less elastic tissue and increased pain. No experts currently recommend this option, although a newer version of it, using the Candela laser, is still used infrequently.

For most patients, there are successful alternatives to surgery, and options should be carefully considered. Even with its high success rates, the use of surgery is still controversial. Since the origins of vestibulitis are still unknown, some doctors don't agree with it. Other health care professionals are using it more frequently because of its high success rate and more immediate results (Bornstein et al. 1995).

Chapter 5

Support and Self-Help for Vulvodynia Sufferers

By Phyllis Mate, President of the National Vulvodynia Association

In 1994, five vulvodynia patients in the Washington, D.C., area decided that they could not possibly be the only ones in the world with vulvodynia. This realization was a significant leap forward for the women because all had suffered for years without receiving a diagnosis, and in some cases had been referred to psychiatrists by physicians who suggested their condition was psychological. Later that year, those five patients made a long-term commitment to become patient advocates by creating the National Vulvodynia Association (NVA). What began as a small support group became a national organization that today serves thousands of women worldwide. We were right—we weren't the only ones!

For many years I was the only one who answered the NVA phone. I've spoken to thousands of women, many of whom shared the same concerns and asked the same questions. What follows are some of the most frequently asked questions and my typical responses. I have a master's degree in clinical psychology, not a medical degree, but have spent a great deal of time studying medical journal articles on vulvodynia and having discussions with vulvodynia experts. Much of what I've learned has resulted from extensive conversations with NVA medical advisory board members including Stanley Marinoff, M.D., director of the Center for Vulvovaginal Disorders in Washington, D.C.; vulvodynia specialist David Foster, M.D., University of Rochester Medical Center; and pain researcher Ursula Wesselmann, M.D., Johns Hopkins University School of Medicine. In editing articles for the NVA newsletter, I have also worked with many other vulvodynia experts including Gae Rodke, M.D., a coauthor of this book, and Elizabeth Stewart, M.D., director of the Stewart-Forbes Vulvovaginal Specialty Service in Boston.

Most Frequently Asked Questions

"Am I going to have this forever?"

That's the hardest question to answer. For some women the condition is chronic and will last years, or possibly "forever." For others, especially those with vestibulitis, there are some success stories. But for both groups it can be a long road from symptom discovery to diagnosis to effective treatment. One of the greatest challenges for women in the earliest stages is coping with the possibility that they may have a chronic condition. Since most women have never heard of vulvodynia before being diagnosed, it's not the same as hearing you have breast cancer or heart disease. With those catastrophic illnesses, you have some idea of what to expect. A diagnosis of vulvodynia initially causes bewilderment as well as anxiety.

"My doctor thinks I may have vulvodynia, but isn't sure. How is it diagnosed?"

Before a diagnosis of vulvodynia is made, sexually transmitted diseases, bacterial or yeast infections, and dermatological diseases must be ruled out. If a patient is diagnosed with another disorder, it must be thoroughly treated first. There is no definitive test for vulvodynia. If symptoms persist after other conditions are eliminated, a diagnosis of vulvodynia is considered. Confirming the diagnosis may be complicated by the possibility that the patient has more than one condition at the same time.

"I've just been diagnosed with vulvodynia. What is the best treatment?"

It may sound self-serving, but in response to this question, I rec-ommend joining the NVA and reading back issues of the newsletters, which contain articles by multiple vulvodynia experts. There is no "best treatment" for vulvodynia, so it's important to inform yourself about all treatment options and discuss them with your gynecologist. In addition to educating yourself and finding a medical professional who is knowledgeable about vulvodynia, it's important to accept that there is no quick fix for this condition. Many patients try several treatment models and discover that a combination of measures works best.

"I have vulvodynia and haven't had sexual relations with my husband for months. Will I ever be able to have sexual intercourse again?"

The goal of treatment is twofold: to relieve pain and to enable the patient to resume pleasurable sexual relations. Vulvodynia symp-toms range from mild to severe. In mild cases, sexual relations may only be slightly affected. In moderate to severe cases, sexual inter-course is difficult, if not impossible. Patients should speak to their gynecologists about measures that can make sexual intercourse com-fortable. Some couples find sex therapy helpful because it teaches and encourages them to engage in forms of physical and sexual inti-macy that are not painful for women with vulvodynia. As treatment progresses and symptoms dissipate, gradual resumption of sexual intercourse is attempted.

"I can't take antidepressants. My doctor prescribed Elavil (amitriptyline), but I stopped it after a week because I couldn't stay awake. What else can I do?"

Call your doctor! When this happens it doesn't necessarily mean you can't tolerate antidepressants. You may need to start at a lower dosage or raise the dosage more slowly. If your problem is waking up in the morning, doctors recommend taking the medication in the early evening instead of at bedtime. Alternately, there are many other antidepressants (and anticonvulsants) that have milder side effects than Elavil. Sometimes you have to try three or four medications (or a combination) before you find the regimen that works best for you and has manageable side effects.

"I've been following my doctor's instructions for a month and my vulvodynia is getting worse. What should I do?"

I've said it above, but it's important enough to repeat, "Call your doctor!" So many patients hesitate to tell their doctor that a treatment isn't working because no one wants to be perceived as a "bad patient." For example, if you're prescribed a topical medication and it burns, call your doctor right away. A little common sense goes a long way—using medication that burns (for vulvar burning!) is probably more harmful than helpful. Many topical creams and ointments contain ingredients that can further irritate vulvar tissue.

"I have had constant burning and pain for months and I'm desperate. How can I stop the pain?"

What I find most distressing in speaking with many sufferers is their passive approach to seeking treatment for pain. They visit their gynecologist and start using ointments, creams, antidepressants, and/or biofeedback, but remain in moderate to severe pain for weeks or months waiting for the treatment to work. If your gynecologist or internist is not comfortable prescribing strong pain-relieving medications on a short-term basis, see a pain specialist. In addition to prescribing medication, a pain specialist may suggest other complementary pain-relieving techniques. Even after vulvar pain is controlled, patients experience flare-ups. If you explain this to a pain specialist, he or she can prescribe effective pain-relieving medication for limited use during flare-ups.

"I have had many yeast infections in the past year that never seem to go away and now I have constant burning. Could I have vulvodynia?"

The main symptoms of a yeast infection are itching and a thick, white discharge, but yeast may also cause burning sensations. The most commonly reported symptom of dysesthetic vulvodynia is burning, although some women also report itching. If you have recurrent yeast infections for many months, you may be at high risk for developing vulvodynia. If you test positive for yeast, be sure to take the full course of antifungal medication your doctor prescribes. (For women with chronic vulvar problems, it is preferable to use oral rather than topical medication.) If yeast symptoms persist, ask your doctor to take another culture. If you've been fully treated for yeast and the culture returns negative, you could have vulvodynia.

"I suffer from urinary difficulties, and sometimes experience vulvar burning. How can I tell if I have vulvodynia?"

Many women suffer from both chronic urinary and vulvar symptoms. For example, the Interstitial Cystitis Association estimates that 25 percent of interstitial cystitis patients suffer from vulvodynia. Because of the location of the urethra and its similarity to vulvar tissue, it may be difficult to discriminate between urinary and vulvar disorders. Even some women with vulvodynia who do not have urinary difficulties report greater discomfort from the pressure of a full bladder. There are some urologists and urogynecologists who are knowledgeable about vulvodynia and going to one of them would be a good place to start.

"Does vaginal childbirth make vulvodynia worse?"

Recently, one of our support group members asked vulvodynia expert Stanley Marinoff, M.D., this question. In the absence of any research in this area, his response was based on many years of clinical experience. According to Dr. Marinoff, most vulvodynia patients who have vaginal deliveries either improve or stay the same and very few get worse. Personally speaking, I know many women with vulvodynia who have had positive experiences with pregnancy and vaginal delivery. (See Gae Rodke's discussion of vulvar pain, pregnancy, and childbirth in chapter 7.)

Patients Helping Patients

The NVA is one of the few established patient advocacy organizations that is run by a volunteer executive director and board of directors. Most services are provided by these individuals or other committed NVA volunteers. The advantage of a patient-run organization is that we have personally experienced both the physical and emotional impact of vulvodynia. This has been a learning process for all of us and our mission is to share what we've learned from our own experiences as well as those of other women.

Information

The more you know about the diagnosis and treatment of chronic vulvar pain, the better-equipped you will be to discuss your options with your doctor. The NVA publishes a newsletter that is read by both patients and medical professionals. Each newsletter contains articles by different medical experts who specialize in treating vulvovaginal pain. Our philosophy is to present all types of medically responsible treatments and encourage patients to discuss the various options with their doctors. The newsletter also answers patients' questions, provides up-to-date information on vulvodynia research studies, and reports on relevant medical conferences, publicity efforts, and progress in our quest for federal funding of vulvodynia research.

In addition to its newsletter, the NVA distributes several thousand informational brochures each year to individual patients, women's health clinics, and medical offices. In the beginning, only vulvovaginal experts requested our patient brochures, but in the past few years, hundreds of ob/gyn practices have asked to receive patient brochures as well as our newsletter. Vulvodynia awareness is spreading! The NVA also maintains a current bibliography of relevant medical journal articles and books that should be helpful to vulvodynia patients.

When you join the NVA by mail or telephone, you receive the most recent newsletter, the bibliography, information on support services, a health survey, and a list of the contents of all previous newsletter issues. If you join on the Web site, www.nva.org, you can order back issues at the same time and they will be included in your new member packet.

Support Services

It is very helpful to speak with other patients about coping with the physical symptoms of vulvodynia and related emotional or sexual issues. The NVA has established a nationwide patient support network and also does its best to provide assistance to women in other countries. Many patients find that speaking to others with vulvodynia is a good source of information and the best way to overcome the emotional isolation that may result from having this disorder. When you join the NVA, you can request the name and contact information for your regional support leader. The vast majority of newly diagnosed patients choose to do so.

Most of our support leaders will communicate with you by telephone or e-mail. In large cities such as New York, Chicago, and Washington, D.C., support groups meet on a monthly or bimonthly basis. Support groups also exist in smaller cities such as Madison, Wisconsin, if enough women express an interest in holding meetings. These groups provide emotional support, host speakers from different medical specialties, and can also raise public awareness through local newspapers or television newscasts. Among the topics discussed at these meetings are how to find medical specialists, treatment options, self-help measures, and dealing with intimate relationships.

Medical Professional Referrals

When the NVA began, our mission was to disseminate information to patients and educate medical professionals, but we did not plan to become a doctor referral service. It quickly became apparent that finding a doctor familiar with the diagnosis and treatment of vulvodynia was a priority for the women who contacted us. In response, we have developed a medical professional database that contains names of vulvodynia experts as well as other doctors, nurse practitioners, and physical therapists who are interested in learning how to treat patients with vulvodynia. If we only listed the vulvodynia specialists nationwide, we probably couldn't generate more than thirty names, and most of these specialists practice in large cities. (If you are able to see a vulvodynia expert, you need to know that they have very busy practices, which makes it very difficult to get a timely appointment. Let the receptionist or nurse know that you are in pain and place your name on their waiting list in the event that there is a cancellation. Call the office every few days to see if there have been any cancellations. Do not assume that someone will call you.)

For women who suspect they have vulvodynia but have not been diagnosed, we often recommend consulting a specialist initially to obtain a diagnosis. This doctor can start you on a treatment regimen or suggest treatment options for you to discuss with your usual gynecologist or other medical professional. When you consult a vulvodynia expert, you can also request that he or she call your gynecologist to discuss your case.

Many women do not live near a vulvodynia expert and can't afford to travel to see one. Consequently, our referral lists include the names of medical professionals who have some familiarity with vulvodynia and receive our newsletters and research updates. The NVA has focused on educating these practitioners and has expanded its professional education services in the past year. Any patient who joins the NVA can have her doctor's name added to our database and we will send our newsletters and other informational materials to his or her office.

Major NVA Initiatives

Educating patients and medical professionals about vulvodynia has been our top priority, but a lot of other work goes on behind the scenes. Publicizing the condition and obtaining federal research funding are two of the areas in which we've made great strides. We're aware of all that remains to be done, but it's gratifying to see that some of our hard work has already made a difference.

Publicizing the Condition

In 1994, print and TV health reporters expressed little interest in covering vulvodynia. It's amazing how much can change in seven years! A few years later, CBS aired a primetime special, *The Body Human*, in which an NVA support group leader, her husband, and her doctor were interviewed about her vestibulectomy. In February 2001, doctors Laura and Jennifer Berman discussed vulvodynia and the NVA on *Oprah*. There have also been dozens of articles on the condition's diagnosis and treatment in popular magazines such as *Redbook*, *Good Housekeeping*, and *Self*.

This past summer, millions of television viewers learned about vulvodynia on the 2001 season premiere of HBO's top-rated show *Sex and the City*. Charlotte, one of the show's main characters, is examined by her gynecologist and told that she may have vulvodynia. She is perplexed when her gynecologist recommends an antidepressant and tells her to keep a daily pain journal. Consistent with the series' lighthearted tone, Charlotte's friends joke about her gynecologist's recommendations at lunch the next day. The NVA received hundreds of phone calls from vulvodynia sufferers who were indignant about the show's unsympathetic portrayal of such a painful condition. The NVA immediately issued a press release praising HBO for tackling the subject, but criticizing its insensitive portrayal. Within the next two weeks, eight major newspapers responded to the release and published articles on the reality of living with vulvodynia.

While the NVA has been working diligently to generate public awareness, we were taken completely by surprise upon the October 2001 release of best-selling author Susanna Kaysen's second memoir, *The Camera My Mother Gave Me*. In this autobiographical account of her desperate search to find treatment for chronic vulvar pain, she writes, "It isn't cancer. It isn't diabetes. It isn't life threatening. It's just horrible" (p. 111). The memoir details both Kaysen's interactions with an extensive number of medical professionals and the wide array of treatments that she tried. I am sure that many vulvodynia sufferers will identify with her seemingly endless frustrating experiences. (Unfortunately, Ms. Kaysen inadvertently made incorrect statements about the NVA in her book. She personally apologized to the NVA in a letter: "I am sorry that I gave the impression that your organization favored or didn't favor certain types of treatment. I didn't intend to misrepresent you, and I know that you are an informational entity, not a prescriptive one.")

Internet Outreach

Shortly after the NVA's formation, cofounder Marjorie MacArthur Veiga promoted the creation of our Web site, www.nva.org. Some board members were skeptical but we trusted her judgment. Marjorie's foresight has enabled us to reach thousands of women worldwide. Most of our medical referrals and support services are concentrated in the U.S., but we also serve hundreds of women in Canada, the U.K., Australia, Israel, and a dozen other countries. In addition to receiving e-mails from women in all fifty states, we have been contacted by women in Malta, India, and Yugoslavia! Regardless of these e-mails' country of origin, their content is universal. Most women write, "I learned so much from your Web site and it's so reassuring to know that you're out there." Another unanticipated result has been the overwhelming number of medical professionals who use our Web site as a resource.

Christin Veasley, my coworker of the past two years, quickly recognized the need to provide information tailored to the needs of medical professionals and is currently working on modifying our site to fulfill this function. In the interim, Christin obtained corporate funding to create a quarterly electronic newsletter summarizing recent medical journal articles on vulvodynia, which we disseminate to interested medical professionals.

Medical Conferences

For many years, the NVA's medical advisory board members have been making clinical and research presentations at meetings of the American College of Obstetricians and Gynecologists (ACOG) and the International Society for the Study of Vulvovaginal Diseases (ISSVD). As the NVA has become more established, we have started coordinating vulvodynia presentations at national medical conferences, including meetings of the American Women's Medical Association and the American Pain Society.

At a recent meeting of ACOG, we were encouraged by the tremendous interest in vulvodynia expressed by the attendees. When these gynecologists visited our booth, we asked them, "Do you treat vulvodynia?" The most frequent reply was, "I try. It's a difficult condition to treat." We were very impressed by their candor as well as their desire to learn more about the condition. Although exhibiting at conferences is expensive, the NVA plans to attend as many as possible. Other than the Internet, it may be the best way for us to reach a large number of medical professionals. By the end of the recent ACOG conference, we had added the names of 500 doctors to our mailing list.

Under the skillful direction of chairperson Maria Turner, M.D., the NVA organized the first National Institutes of Health (NIH) vulvodynia workshop in April 1997. More than 200 medical specialists from all over the world met to discuss the current state of knowledge of vulvodynia and to determine future research strategies. This workshop was a turning point because it eventually led to the first federal funding of vulvodynia research. The next NIH vulvodynia symposium for medical professionals is scheduled for spring 2003, and NVA medical advisory board member Dr. Ursula Wesselmann and I are members of the planning committee.

Lobbying for Research Funding

After the first NIH conference, the NVA approached Peter Reinecke, legislative director for U.S. Senator Tom Harkin, Democrat of Iowa, because the senator was a well-known women's health advocate. All of us are indebted to Senator Harkin and Mr. Reinecke for championing our cause and ensuring that vulvodynia has been included in Congress's NIH appropriations reports. Ironically, some members of the U.S. Congress learned about vulvodynia before some medical professionals did! The most recent Senate NIH appropriations report contained the following language: "Preliminary new research indicates that millions of American women suffer from vulvodynia, a painful and often debilitating disorder of the female reproductive system. Since fiscal year 1998, the Committee has called on the National Institute of Child Health and Human Development (NICHD) to support research on the prevalence, causes, and treatment of vulvodynia. The Committee urges NICHD to significantly expand research on vulvodynia."

Largely as a result of congressional pressure, the NICHD allocated $1 million per year for five years for vulvodynia research and funded the first four studies in early 2001. By the end of the year, an additional vulvodynia research proposal received funding. NICHD's interest in researching the condition is growing and should be significantly advanced by the upcoming 2003 NIH symposium. One of the first proposals funded was a prevalence study by epidemiologist Bernard Harlow, Ph.D., and gynecologist Elizabeth Stewart, M.D., both of Harvard University. This five-year project will determine the prevalence of chronic vulvar pain among American women and differentiate its various subsets. According to Dr. Harlow, the study's preliminary data suggests that 18 percent of American women have suffered from chronic vulvar discomfort in their lifetime. Contrary to previous estimates that were in the hundreds of thousands, it appears that millions of American women suffer from some type of vulvodynia.

NVA Research Fund

The NIH typically funds researchers who submit scientifically sound proposals with promising pilot data. The purpose of the NVA Research Fund is to pay for pilot studies, enabling researchers to collect the data they need to receive substantial NIH funding. The pilot studies chosen are those that will advance knowledge of the causes of vulvodynia and also have potential to lead to more effective treatment. The NVA's first research award recipient, neurologist Ursula Wesselmann, M.D., of the Johns Hopkins University School of Medicine, recently received NIH funding to study the neurophysiological mechanisms of pain associated with vaginal inflammation. In 2002, Dr. Wesselmann will begin an NVA-funded pilot study examining hormonal effects on dysesthetic vulvodynia in post-menopausal women. Other recipients of NVA research grants have submitted proposals to NIH that are currently being reviewed.

Self-Help Tips

While seeking effective treatment for vulvar pain, here are some coping measures to help relieve symptoms and prevent further irritation. Even when your symptoms are under control, you should continue using some of these measures to prevent a recurrence or flare-up.

Clothing and Laundry

You may have to purchase a few new clothing items. First on the list should be all-white cotton underwear, a recommendation that applies to all women. Most vulvodynia sufferers are more comfortable wearing skirts or loose-fitting pants. Tight pants and pantyhose, in particular, should be avoided. Long skirts are especially useful because they can eliminate the need for pantyhose, which creates friction and increases moisture in the vulvar area. Purchase pairs of thigh highs or knee-high hose instead. Additionally, to keep moisture to a minimum, remove your wet bathing suit promptly after swimming. If you can find one, buy a cotton bathing suit or sew a piece of cotton inside your nylon bathing suit. To wash your clothing, use a dermatologically approved, unscented detergent such as Purex or Clear. Double rinse your underwear and any other garments that come in contact with the vulva, and do not use fabric softener on any undergarments.

Personal Hygiene

Gynecologists recommend washing the vulva with water only because soap can be very irritating to the delicate tissue. During bathing or showering, avoid getting soap, shampoo, or any scented products on the vulvar area. Some women find adding Aveeno to their bathwater very soothing; do not use bubble bath or bath oil. Always avoid the use of feminine hygiene products, including sprays, powders, and perfumed creams. If you are experiencing a flare-up, using a lukewarm or cool sitz bath three times per day may be helpful. Sitz baths are available at local drug stores for about thirty dollars. Please note: Do not overdo your hygiene practice: washing too often or too vigorously can make this condition worse.

Some women who have vulvodynia experience problems with urination. Obviously, you should use the softest, unscented white toilet paper available (e.g., Charmin Ultra). Some women find wiping after urination, even with the softest toilet paper, very uncomfortable. In this case, you can fill a small squirt bottle with cool to lukewarm water and rinse the vulva after urinating, and gently pat the area dry or use the low/cool setting on your blow-dryer. Additionally, the more dilute the urine is, the less vulvar irritation it causes, so drink at least eight glasses of water a day.

During menstruation, use only 100 percent cotton menstrual pads and tampons (e.g., Glad Rags). Avoid super-thin maxipads as they contain irritating moisture-absorbing chemicals. Any thick pad can also cause problems, as dried blood can be irritating. Opt for minipads (Light Days is a good, easily accessible option) and change them often. Try not to use mini pads for non-menstrual discharge; instead, change your underwear as often as necessary. As for tampons, slender and regular non-scented versions are best for you. Some women find the tampon string irritates tender vulvar skin. You can curb irritation by coating the string with Vaseline. Change tampons often to reduce the build up of harmful bacteria.

Diet

Many women have read on the Internet or heard from their doctors that there may be a link between diet and vulvar pain symptoms. The idea of being helped by simply modifying one's diet is very appealing. Consequently, almost every patient I've talked to has tried the low-oxalate diet and calcium citrate (see chapter 4). Based on the NVA's survey, it seems that about 15 percent obtain modest relief from this regimen. I don't necessarily recommend it, but I don't discourage people from trying it either. You should be aware that some health professionals consider it an unhealthy diet, especially during pregnancy. If you've been on the low-oxalate and calcium citrate regimen for six months and your symptoms haven't improved significantly, it's time to try another treatment!

The low-oxalate diet aside, some women observe that eating a certain food aggravates their symptoms. For example, foods that are high in acidic content, such as citrus fruits and tomatoes, sometimes cause a problem. One way to deal with this difficulty is to drink more water and dilute the urine, but if you find that eating a certain food consistently increases your pain level, try eliminating it from your diet.

Drinking a lot of water can also help prevent constipation, which some women report exacerbates vulvar symptoms. Another way to prevent constipation is to eat a high-fiber diet that nutritional experts say is beneficial to your health anyway. Good sources of fiber are bran cereals, vegetables, fruits, and even popcorn! (One of the practical problems with the low-oxalate diet is that it eliminates many high-fiber foods.) If you're taking moderate to high doses of tricyclic antidepressants, such as amitriptyline or desipramine, you may need to take Metamucil and/or Colace to maintain regularity.

Over-the-Counter Medications

If you are considering the use of any over-the-counter topical medications, consult your doctor first. Sometimes these products' additives and preservatives cause irritation. Your doctor may recommend a pharmacy that can prepare a topical medication using a base that is much less irritating than over-the-counter preparations.

If you are experiencing an abnormal amount of vaginal discharge and suspect that you have an infection, make an appointment with your doctor or nurse practitioner immediately. An increase in vaginal discharge usually further irritates the vulva. Do not self-treat! Wait for the results of a vaginal culture before using any over-the-counter or prescription medications. Antifungals and antibiotics can disrupt the delicate balance of flora in the vagina, so it's not wise to use any of these medications if you have not been diagnosed with an infection.

Sexual Relationships

By far the most important thing to do when experiencing pain during intercourse is to tell your partner and stop immediately. Having intercourse to please your partner even though you're in pain can be both physically damaging and harmful to your relationship. This doesn't mean that you have to stop having intercourse indefinitely! Until your symptoms are under control, try to find other ways to express affection and be sexually intimate with your partner. After you find a treatment that alleviates some or all of your pain and you feel ready to resume sexual intercourse, there are some measures that are helpful. Always use a lubricant that is water soluble, for example Astroglide (not K-Y jelly or Vaseline). Do not use contraceptive creams, especially spermicides, for they are extremely irritating to sensitive tissue. You may also find that certain positions are more comfortable than others.

Women with vulvar vestibulitis, in particular, may require a topical anesthetic such as Lidocaine to use prior to intercourse. Lidocaine 5 percent is a prescription medication that is applied to the vestibule and may sting slightly for the first few minutes after application. Before you attempt to use a prescribed anesthetic on the vulva, you can try it on another area of your body, such as your inner thigh. If it isn't uncomfortable except for some initial stinging, apply a thin layer to the vestibule (but not right before intercourse the first time). If you do not have a negative reaction, then you should try using it about five minutes prior to intercourse. After intercourse, doctors recommend urinating to prevent a urinary tract infection and rinsing the vulva with cool to lukewarm water to minimize irritation. If you experience pain after intercourse, apply a frozen gel pack or ice wrapped in a soft towel for ten to fifteen minutes. You can purchase a gel pack at any drugstore and keep it in the freezer. Never apply ice or a cold pack directly to the vulva. As an alternative, some women experience relief using a sitz bath filled with cool water.

Physical Exercise

In spite of your condition, there are reasons why you should try to continue some kind of exercise program. First, it is beneficial for your overall physical and mental health, and second, there is scientific evidence that aerobic exercise increases the amount of endorphins (natural painkillers) circulating in the body. The challenge is finding a type of exercise that is comfortable for you. Obviously, you should avoid horseback riding and bicycle riding because they apply direct pressure to the vulva, although you can buy modified bicycle seats that eliminate the problem. Swimming may or may not work because the chlorine in pools can be irritating for vulvodynia sufferers. Some women find that they can swim in the ocean or a lake, but not in a pool.

Avoid exercises that create a lot of friction and moisture in the vulvar area. Instead, try lower intensity exercises such as walking. I know women who've had such severe pain that they couldn't walk at all in the beginning. After a few months of treatment, many of these women are walking thirty minutes five times a week. If you experience additional discomfort after exercise, try a cool to lukewarm sitz bath or apply a cold pack wrapped in a towel for fifteen minutes. During severe flare-ups, it's probably wise to temporarily suspend your exercise program.

There are many different ways to exercise. A growing body of evidence suggests that yoga has beneficial effects on individuals with chronic health conditions. It is also widely accepted that stress can exacerbate pain, so you may want to learn relaxation exercises and other pain control methods. Check out *The Relaxation and Stress Reduction Workbook* (Davis, Eshelman, and McKay 2000) or *The Chronic Pain Control Workbook* (Catalano and Hardin 1996).

Keeping a Journal

Many psychologists and medical professionals advocate keeping a journal as a way to understand and cope with vulvar pain. They recommend rating your pain level on a scale from 0 to 5 every day. As you try new therapies, record them in your journal. Keeping track of your pain level will enable you to evaluate whether a particular treatment is helping you. Additionally, expressing your feelings and describing your experience with vulvodynia can be emotionally therapeutic.

Here is how journal writing helps Anne, age 29:

I began a personal journal in early 1992 shortly after my husband and I became engaged. At that time, I was having frequent yeast infections and intermittent mild pain, yet my condition had not been diagnosed. My early writing reflected events in my life, as well as my feelings about finishing graduate school and embarking on a new career. It was a stressful period for me, and my physician suggested that my pain and yeast infections were due to

*stress. When my condition worsened, and the pain became
a continual burning, I was referred to another doctor who
diagnosed me immediately. He also confirmed that I
wasn't the only woman suffering from this condition.*

*My writings reflected my anger and frustration about
how long my symptoms had existed and apparently would
continue. Then things became even worse. I couldn't
engage in many of the activities I used to enjoy, my work
was disrupted by the pain, and there were increased
tensions between my husband and myself. During this
period, I was constantly in and out of the doctor's office
and given all kinds of medications to try.*

*Since vulvodynia is not easy to talk about, I found
myself turning to my journal with increasing frequency. It
was a way to unburden myself without worrying about
someone passing judgment on me. Sometimes I was so low
I didn't know how I'd get through the day. In one entry I
described my physical appearance (recent weight loss,
dark circles under my eyes, graying hair) and how I felt
old, tired, and completely undesirable. I wrote, "Why
me?" and "Will I ever be normal again?" An especially
low point occurred when my husband and I started seeing
a therapist, and both of them pressured me to take
antidepressant medication. As a health care professional
myself, I was embarrassed that I needed that kind of help.
I resisted initially, but eventually began taking Zoloft.
Looking back on my writings at that time, it is clear that I
was very angry and felt as though my husband and
therapist were ganging up on me. But several months
later, journal entries reveal I was feeling somewhat better
and beginning to regain some energy. This renewed energy
helped me to continue my struggle with vulvodynia.*

*Keeping a journal may not work for everyone, but it
was beneficial for me. Today when I read my old entries,
they remind me of a dark and scary period in my life. But
they also help me to see how far I've come. If I have a
setback now, I pull out my writings to remind me that my
life isn't nearly as dreadful now as it was then. My journal
also gives me hope that someday I will be able to make*

some sense out of this physically and emotionally painful condition.

Work and Everyday Living

The most common practical issues in the workplace for vulvodynia sufferers are how to dress comfortably and how to sit comfortably most of the day. If your occupation requires sitting for extended periods of time, try using a donut. You can cover it with a pillowcase or a slipcover, so it looks like a chair cushion. Also, find a way to intersperse sitting with periods of standing. For example, arrange your office so that you can stand while you're on the phone. Women with vulvodynia also have to deal with the issue of whether to discuss their condition with their coworkers or employer. This is obviously a personal choice and if you're not comfortable discussing it, you can always say you need to stand up and move around because you have back pain.

When you're relaxing at night, you can read or watch television lying on the couch or in a recliner. You may have already found that some chairs in your home are more comfortable than others. If you haven't already discovered it yourself, there are a few issues to consider in selecting a car. Obviously you want a car with a smooth ride, but if you're considering leather car seats, beware that they get very hot in the sun.

A Final Word

The best advice I can give to you is to seek treatment promptly, consult a vulvodynia specialist if possible, educate yourself (and your ob/gyn), see a pain specialist if needed, and speak openly with your significant other about the difficulties of living with vulvodynia. Most importantly, do not give up. The women who are assertive and persistent in seeking treatment usually achieve the most successful outcomes.

For More Information

NVA
P.O. Box 449
Silver Spring, MD 02914-4491
301-299-0775
www.nva.org

Chapter 6

Managing Your Chronic Pain

As someone with vulvodynia, you suffer with chronic pain—that is, long-lasting, intense pain that is persistent or comes in episodes and negatively affects your functioning or well-being. You may not realize that a lot of research has been done on chronic pain—and much of it may be helpful as you learn to manage your own. Other common chronic pain ailments are arthritis, joint injuries, and fibromyalgia. More than 37 million Americas live with chronic pain every day (Pollin 1995).

The vast majority of people who deal with chronic pain describe their condition as out of control (Sanders and Mate 1998). Even though there are places they can go for help—pain management specialists in particular—68 percent of sufferers never seek help. Even more alarming, they are never even referred to pain management clinics or specialists. As a result, patients float from doctor to doctor looking for help. More than half switch physicians at least once. One-fourth of all sufferers have been to three or more doctors in search of relief. People with chronic pain tend to be unhappy with their health care providers' lack of knowledge about pain and the general unwillingness to treat it aggressively.

Many suffer in silence. Chronic pain patients—including vulvodynia victims—slowly give up parts of their lives in search of comfort. For example, women may find they no longer exercise because tight pants hurt their vulvas. Some can't get proper amounts of sleep. Still others find that they no longer work, socialize, or have fulfilling sex lives. It is no wonder that some patients wind up with a terrible side effect of their chronic pain. They wind up depressed.

Treat Your Chronic Pain and Take It Seriously

Depression may result from having chronic pain. For some, it's manageable. For others, it's serious. For one woman, depression due to vulvodynia was deadly. In a well-known case, an English woman, Yvonne Wallis, committed suicide in her late forties after suffering from severe vulvodynia for eighteen months. She was only forty-seven when her pain began. She believed that her symptoms were associated with a prescription cream she used to cure a yeast infection. After being in terrible pain, her doctor told her she was having a severe reaction and the discomfort would go away within the week. It did not go away. She saw specialists but got no relief. Wallis wasn't able to sleep or move around normally, and she was taking sleeping pills and painkillers regularly. In his book, her son Mark Wallis wrote, "She would hold my arms, crying and saying that she could not take any more and that no one was helping her. When I would hold her, I felt her whole body twitch with pain" (Wallis 1996).

Yvonne Wallis had the support of her family, but she didn't know anyone else with her problem. In fact, she didn't know much about vulvodynia at all. Wallis was in a rural community without access to the latest research, or even to doctors who were aware of the disorder. She spiraled into a cycle of severe depression. Although proper psychological treatment might have saved her life, neither her family nor her doctors knew enough about chronic pain to help her.

Thankfully, most women won't become suicidal because of vulvodynia. But the vast majority will find themselves depressed or anxious at times. No matter what level of depression you experience due to your chronic pain, realize that there is help for you. Pain management specialists, including psychologists, are available to help you get your life back.

Dealing with Depression

People who experience any kind of chronic pain experience bouts of depression. The following stories are from two women who explain how they cope with the lows that are very real, routine parts of their lives.

"I Get By with Support from My Friends and Family"

I am a thirty-one-year-old long-term sufferer of vulvodynia. But for the past two years, I have been virtually pain-free, without burning. That was until two weeks ago, when my vulvodynia flared up while I was sitting at my work desk. I became filled with anxiety, fearful that it had returned permanently. I waited a few days and called the pain management clinic. My unique, supportive doctor of the past three years calmed me down, assured me that symptoms fluctuate, and suggested that I would probably improve in a few days. He also let me know that if I didn't feel any better, there were plenty of alternatives to reduce the intense pain.

I attended my regularly scheduled support group meeting, which I look forward to each month. We discussed our fears about flare-ups and reminded each other that flare-ups come and go. By the time the meeting ended, I felt better.

My family called often during this period and that was a source of great comfort to me. With all of the emotional support from my family and NVA [National Vulvodynia Association] friends, I survived this flare-up and am back to feeling like my usual self. Support is great medicine to aid recovery!

"I Talk to Friends with Vulvodynia"

I have had vulvodynia for the past four years, and I can truthfully say that today I feel 90 percent better than I did when it started. In fact, most of the time I feel no discomfort from it. I have found a combination of treatments that works very well for me. Once in a while, however, the pain flares up for no apparent reason. I always feel frustrated when this happens, and I start to get very anxious, wondering if I will be able to stop the pain. These episodes bring back memories of what it was like in the beginning, when I knew nothing about vulvodynia except that it caused terrible pain.

The first thing I do during a flare-up is call one of my friends with vulvodynia. No one can reassure me as much as a fellow sufferer. My friend reminds me that we have both been down this road before and have always bounced back to a comfortable place. Often, humor works its way into our conversation, and we move on to other topics, reminding me that I am much more than a woman with a chronic pain disorder. At least I am in control of what it does to my mind, if not always my body.

Modify Your Thinking

Cut yourself, and others in your life, some slack! Pain may make you irritable, but you don't always realize it. Maybe your friends and family are suffering from chronic pain, too. Remember that you are not the only one who has ever felt like this. It is natural for chronic pain sufferers to believe that their pain is the worst. But many others have pain, too. It is good to keep this in perspective.

How Do Your Loved Ones Handle Your Pain?

Chronic pain causes the dynamics of your relationships to change. Friends may not see you as much because you have quit the morning walking club, or perhaps you aren't sleeping well, so you're too tired for happy hour. Family members may notice your changes and irritability. The person who is most profoundly affected, besides you of course, is your spouse. Not only is he forced to watch you suffer—which is never easy for him—he is also dealing with huge changes in the nature of your relationship. You may not be able to do as many daily tasks as you used to; you may not be as devoted to your work anymore; and you may simply not be able to engage in sexual intercourse. While he wants to be supportive and help you, he probably wishes things could be like they used to be, too. Vulvodynia becomes a serious issue for both of you. How do you handle it?

Irene Pollin in *Taking Charge* (1995) suggests,

> If your spouse is reluctant to express emotions, don't push. . . . You can still explain that even though you understand his restraint, you need to cope by confronting your feelings. You may feel disappointed that your [spouse] doesn't communicate the way you do, but don't underestimate [his] feelings. Even though the means of expression differ, they may be as strong as yours. Aware of the disparity, you can seek help from support groups, friends, and other extended family members.

In short, if your spouse—like most—tries to understand your pain but sometimes just doesn't "get it," develop a support group of friends, family, and health care professionals whom you can talk to. Or contact the NVA to find out whether there is already a group in your area or to get help in starting one.

Do You Tell Others About Your Vulvodynia?

One woman, thirty-four, writes:

I decided to tell only my closest friends in addition to my husband. Since most of my close friends are women, that minimized the embarrassment. Most women have had yeast infections, so they can relate to the symptoms. I found that once I told one person, it was easier the next time. But it's definitely more difficult to reveal that one has chronic vulvar pain than it would be to discuss chronic back pain.

I also have found that people who have not experienced chronic pain do not understand how debilitating it can be. There is the erroneous belief that one can always minimize the pain by not thinking about it. Many people don't realize that the ability to distract oneself varies with the severity of the pain.

I used to have difficulty telling the men I dated about this unusual problem. Some of my boyfriends thought I was sexually uptight because I had pain in the clitoral area, and I never really tried to explain it because I didn't know what it was myself. Twenty years ago when I first started dating, doctors didn't even have a name for it. Now my husband understands that my pain is real and that other women have this disorder.

I would like to be able to tell more people that I have vulvodynia. After all, the public has learned to talk openly about prostate disease, breast cancer, and sexually transmitted diseases. And medication for vaginal yeast infections is advertised constantly on television. So why should it be taboo to talk about vulvar pain? As with other uncomfortable subjects, the more we are willing to talk about vulvodynia, the easier it will be to deal with.

Gender and Chronic Pain

Many researchers believe that men and women experience chronic pain differently—and recent studies are proving this to be the case. The following findings were reported in the *NVA News* (Sanders and Mate 1998).

1. **When in pain: Men are grumpier than women.** Researcher Francis Keefe, Ph.D., of Ohio University compared male and female coping abilities and emotional behavior in a coed group of arthritis sufferers. She found that women use more coping strategies than men, and men were more likely to be in bad moods as a result of pain. Women seem to have more control over the negative emotional consequences of being in pain.

2. **Women are better sympathizers.** When Keefe judged patients' ability to rate his or her spouse's pain, she found

that women were much more accurate than men in evaluating their partner's pain.

3. **Painkillers don't work the same in males and females.** Ursula Wesselmann, M.D., of Johns Hopkins University Medical School, reported that pain management drugs useful in men with testicular pain (including some antidepressants and anticonvulsants) were less effective in women with pelvic pain. Other recent studies have found that nonsteroidal and anti-inflammatories (e.g., ibuprofen) are less effective for treating chronic pain in women, but that certain opioids are more effective. Wesselmann proposes that studies comparing different medications for pelvic pain syndrome and vulvodynia are greatly needed and will lead to better treatment strategies.

4. **Male/female differences in chronic pain perception.** Scientist Jeffrey Mogil, Ph.D., performed experiments on mice indicating that genetics accounted for differences in pain perception between males and females. Several recent studies suggest that certain sex hormones, such as estrogen and testosterone, may explain why women experience pain more intensely than men. Pain researcher Serge Marchard, Ph.D., of the University of Quebec, proposes that testosterone seems to be protective against pain, while estrogen makes females more vulnerable to pain.

Does Anyone Have Time for This Pain?

If we look at vulvodynia as a pain disorder, we can gain new perspective on ways to treat it. Vulvar pain is often due to gynecological or dermatological conditions. The most important medical society specializing in these conditions is the International Society for the Study of Vulvovaginal Disease, established as an interdisciplinary group with common interests in working to study and treat various conditions afflicting women. Until recently (1993) this group was made up of gynecologists, dermatologists, and pathologists from around the world. More recently, psychologists and a physical therapist have become members, a process which involves presenting research in relevant topics, including vulvar pain syndromes. Hopefully, researchers in neurology and pain management will direct their knowledge to study vulvar pain and join in this important work. Collaboration with researchers who deal with chronic pain (in various areas of the body) could prove fruitful.

Obviously, a more integrated approach is necessary. While gynecologists and dermatologists must continue to diagnose and treat vulvar skin problems and infections, they also need to be aware of the biological, psychological, and functional rehabilitative approaches to treating vulvodynia that make up chronic pain management.

Pain management in general has long been a major challenge to the traditional field of Western medicine. When it comes to pain relief, modern health specialists are trained to rely heavily on pharmaceuticals. To be more effective in treating pain, doctors should rely not only on medications but also focus on other possible contributing issues, even if the causes are still unknown. By incorporating a variety of traditional and alternative healing modalities to correct the source of the chronic pain, the symptoms may be more successfully reduced or alleviated.

Ways You Can Ease Your Chronic Pain

Suffering is greatly affected by what patients believe about their own pain. Too often, sufferers hold on to ideas that work against them and increase their misery. Look at these following negative (untrue) thoughts. Then read on to get more facts about chronic pain.

Common Fictions

1. Pain always means something is wrong physically.

2. If your pain can't be explained, something is wrong with you.

3. Some people don't want to get better.

4. The doctor knows more about your vulvar pain than you do.

5. If you complain a lot, you are a weak, bad patient.

6. Not complaining about pain will make it go away.

7. If a cure can't be found, you'll just have to learn to live with pain.

Pain Does Not Always Mean Something Is Wrong Physically

As we have learned in previous chapters, vulvar pain frequently starts with some kind of physical irritation or trauma such as an infection or allergic reaction. This initial phase of pain is called acute pain, it serves as a warning signal, and it usually resolves quickly with prompt treatment (as in a yeast infection). This is not the kind of pain people fret about most. Instead, patients worry about ongoing or chronic pain. Chronic discomfort, by definition, is pain that persists beyond the usual healing time. The problem is that while the pain persists, other problems in addition to the initial source of pain arise. Those problems include muscle tension, changes in circulation, postural imbalances, and changes in the functioning of the central nervous system.

The exact causes of chronic pain are not fully understood, but we do know that unrelieved pain is associated with increased metabolism, increase in brain activity, changes in blood circulation in the brain, and changes in the limbic-hypothalmic system (the part of the brain that's responsible for emotions).

Pain is also a subjective experience. It involves your mind and your emotions, as well as your body. For example, think of how you can remember what pain felt like yesterday, and you can certainly anticipate what pain might feel like tomorrow. In this way, pain is a thought process. It involves a range of feelings including fear, anxiety, and depression. Why? Because people automatically associate sensations of discomfort with something unpleasant such as a severe injury or with a situation in which they were in real, immediate danger. This response is automatic and natural—but it does work to exaggerate human worries concerning pain.

It's important to realize that thinking about pain in purely physical terms is inadequate and misleading. Often, pain isn't as intense or uncomfortable as we thought it would be. If we know we aren't in danger, that the pain is not a sign of immediate risk, and that it will wane (and sometimes wax!), we can at least feel less threatened and avoid all of the unpleasant reactions that fear adds to the way we feel.

If Your Pain Can't Be Explained, You Should Still Take It Seriously

The sad truth is that there are many occasions when medical care providers just can't find out why certain patients experience discomfort. At some time or another, most vulvar pain patients have been told that there is no adequate medical explanation for their complaints. Unfortunately, the doctor—and even the patient herself—may believe her problem is psychological in origin. Next, the physician may imply that the pain is somehow not real—and inadvertently increase the suffering. For the record, the pain does exist; it is real; it is not in your head. Doctors don't know everything yet, and much pain research still remains to be done.

As an example of this thinking, let's look at a recent study of Americans with lower back pain. No adequate medical explanation for the patient's pain could be found in the majority of 10,000 cases (Gatchel et al. 1995). Unfortunately, many professionals (who truthfully should know better) use this lack of an explanation as an excuse to blame the patient for his or her own pain. Interestingly, the words "malingering" and "secondary gain" are often attached to patients with unexplained pain who have failed to respond to treatment.

The reality is that chronic discomfort is a complex personal experience. Someone once defined pain as follows: It is "whatever the experiencing person says it is, whenever the experiencing person says it does." The point is that, yes, you may have to learn to cope with pain without knowing why it exists. Dealing with that is difficult enough. Patients can't let other people add unnecessary guilt to their already complicated lives. Patients also have to make sure they get psychological support when they need it, including therapy and medication if needed.

You Do Want to Get Better

Frustrated health care professionals commonly express the idea that people don't want to get better, for whatever reason. They point to what they call patient "secondary gain," which is medical jargon for any benefit a sufferer obtains from her pain. Physicians (and sometimes people close to the sufferer like employers and even family members) point to the attention and assistance a pain patient gets due to limited activity or functional capacity. This way of thinking is unfair. Research shows it is extremely rare for patients to exaggerate pain. Sometimes sufferers are unfairly accused of laziness as well. Reasonableness in requesting accommodations will go a long way to heading off this attitude. When you must request a change in work responsibilities, for example, try to think of something *you* could do to lighten others' loads in return. Offer before anyone asks you for assistance. That way, you get some choice in your tasks, and you have more bargaining power.

The Doctor Does Not Necessarily Know More About Your Vulvar Pain Than You Do

According to some alarming statistics, chronic pain is "grossly undertreated" in most patients. In a recent, somewhat shocking survey, 50 percent of chronic pain patients believed their pain relief was inadequate, and they had considered suicide to escape their discomfort (Hitchcock, Ferrel, and McCaffery 1994).

What are the reasons for the widespread lack of pain treatment? It is probably due to pain relief being a low priority in our current health care system, a lack of real knowledge about pain management among health care professionals and patients, and because patients tend to underreport their pain—possibly because they worry about cultural and social backlash if they do complain. (You can control how you are treated, to a degree, by modifying your behavior. Instead of whining or complaining, always be firm and professional.)

To assume that all treatment options have been explored is a huge mistake, particularly if you are still experiencing intolerable pain. You are the only one who really knows what your pain is like. Don't be afraid to exercise your rights as a consumer. Find a professional who is willing to try many new treatments to help you be comfortable in your everyday life.

You Have a Right to Complain! (Just Try to Do It Constructively)

Most chronic pain sufferers feel trapped and helpless; they are sick of how they feel and don't want to burden anyone else with their seemingly unsolvable problems. They think there's no point talking about their pain because it won't help anyway. Unfortunately, these ideas often lead to silence concerning their pain when seeking medical help. Without speaking up, medications aren't prescribed, treatments aren't explored, and the patient winds up with unnecessary frustration and anguish. Pain is invisible and subjective—no one can know what it is like unless the patient speaks up. So it is vital that you, as a sufferer, describe exactly how you feel and how pain affects you. Whoever treats you is totally reliant on the information you provide. So be honest with your doctor! If there are reasons you feel you can't or won't be able to do what the doctor suggests, speak up. Perhaps there is another choice or a way to modify the regimen to address your concerns. Perhaps the doctor needs to convince and reassure you that his treatments are your best options. But if you don't speak up, it's you who loses.

Not Complaining About Pain Will Not Make It Go Away

Some patients have thought, "Pain is unconscious," or "I'm the only one with this terrible, unbelievable pain." False. Many, maybe even most, people have a chronic painful condition or limitation. No one talks about it, feeling that they are alone or may be discriminated against if they speak up. Sometimes this limits even the sufferer's ability to sympathize with others who complain or request special accommodations.

If a Cure Can't Be Found, You Do Not Just Have to Learn to Live with Pain

With a few rare exceptions, there is no need for anybody to have to live with unbearable pain today. There are more treatment options available than ever before, ranging from advanced medical procedures to alternative therapies. Take advantage of the latest research and techniques!

Treatment Options to Help Alleviate Chronic Pain

Let's go over the range of treatments available for chronic pain. Why? Because other therapies that have been used for chronic pain in other body systems could prove useful for vulvodynia patients (even though there is still very little published literature on the use of these treatments for vulvar pain).

The most common medical pain management procedures often involve multimodal approaches. The literature suggests that combining several different pain treatments can provide effective pain relief. In addition, using small amounts of various medications can enhance the benefits while minimizing the side effects. Effective management of vulvar pain may involve health care practitioners from several different disciplines.

Pharmaceutical and Surgical Treatments

The most common, traditional medical pain management therapies are outlined in the following list. For a more thorough discussion of how some of these may help you with your vulvodynia, refer to chapter 4.

Membrane-Stabilizing Oral Medications (or Nerve-Stabilizing Medications)

Both tricyclic antidepressants like amitriptyline (Elavil), nortriptyline (Pamelor), and anticonvulsants such as gabapentin (Neurontin) or carbamazepine (Tegretol) have been reported to be effective.

Non-Steroidal Anti-Inflammatories (NSAIDs)

Unfortunately, drugs like ibuprofen (Advil) and naproxen (Aleve) have not been helpful in vulvar pain except for their non-specific pain relief effects.

Regional Sympathetic Blockade (or Injecting Local Anesthetics into Tissue)

Pain research suggests that regional sympathetic blockade (also called lumbar sympathetic block, stellate ganglion block, and intravenous regional block) is effective in providing relief from some forms of chronic pain. Questions remain regarding adverse health effects such as hypotension, hyperalgesia, and sensory or motor problems. The literature on the use of pudendal or hypogastric nerve blockade in the treatment of vulvar pain disorders is limited. Due to the disconcerting numbness and possible negative effects on bowel and bladder function—as well as the possibility of "uneven" blockade with "windows," or areas, not relieved being even more distracting by comparison to the numb areas—this technique may be of limited usefulness in vulvar pain.

Corticosteroid (Steroid) Injection Therapy

Although research suggests that topical corticosteroids in the form of creams or ointments could be useful in improving pain and enhancing patient functioning and quality of life, more recent research shows that topical corticosteroids may not in fact be so useful. Locally injected corticosteroids are effective in providing pain relief for some chronic pain syndromes in various parts of the body. However, there are no studies on the effectiveness of locally injected corticosteroids in treatment of vulvar pain.

Neurostimulation Therapy (or Electronic Nerve Stimulation)

Research supports the use of transcutaneous electrical nerve stimulation (TENS) and spinal cord stimulation (SCS) techniques in providing relief of chronic pain in several conditions, including low back pain. These techniques seem to provide the same relief as peripheral nerve stimulation (PNS) techniques. The possible side effects of TENS, PNS, and SCS are unclear. There is no reported literature on the use of these techniques in the treatment of vulvar pain disorders.

Opioid Therapy (or Narcotic Pain Medication)

Opioid therapy for chronic pain management may be administered in several different ways. The most common is systemic delivery (e.g., oral, transdermal patches, or intravenously with injections or IVs). Opioids also may be delivered directly to the neural roots or spinal chord (i.e., epidural, intrathecal infection). Research supports the analgesic usefulness of systemic opioids. However, the literature suggests that systemic use of opioids may be associated with harmful effects such as increased need for larger doses, addiction, itching, nausea, constipation, decreased mental acuity, and respiratory depression. There are no reports in the medical literature specifically relating to the use of opioids in the treatment of vulvar pain.

Note: Narcotics should be a last-resort treatment for vulvodynia patients. They do not improve your condition; instead they deaden symptoms. (And these drugs reduce your ability to feel pleasurable sensations as well as painful ones.) In addition, narcotics can remove sufferers' motivation to pursue other, better therapies.

Neuroablative Techniques (or Removal of Neural Tissue)

Neuroablative techniques destroy neural tissue using chemicals such as alcohol or phenol, or using thermal lesion techniques such as freezing or radiofrequency. Research suggests that chemical and thermal neuroablative techniques can provide some control of chronic pain. Severe adverse health effects from treatment are possible but rarely reported. There is no medical literature on the use of neuroablative techniques in the treatment of essential vulvar pain disorders. The long-term side effects should be carefully considered. They include numbness, muscle weakness, and sexual or urinary dysfunction. There is also the chance of worsening the pain if neural tissue is not completely destroyed. In vulvar pain patients in particular, increased trauma to the area may even *cause* the problem or keep it going.

Alternative Therapies

Along with traditional medical pain management approaches used by specialized pain anesthesiologists, neurologists, and psychiatrists, a large number of complementary medical therapies are now being used to treat chronic pain disorders. We covered some of these in chapter 4, but have summarized all the alternatives in the following list.

Homeopathic Therapy

Homeopathy is a unique technique for treating disease. Substances that produce disease-like symptoms are administered in tiny doses. Some patients report relief, but since homeopathy is tailored to the individual, no two patients are likely to get exactly the same treatment. This makes evaluating the effectiveness of homeopathy difficult.

Allergy and Sensitivity Elimination

Allergies are defined as an abnormally high sensitivity to certain substances or microorganisms. Common signs of allergy include itching and irritating skin rashes. In many vulvar pain patients, allergies or sensitivities to soaps, feminine hygiene products, and laundry detergents may add to vulvar irritation. In patients with histories of allergies, thorough investigation and effective treatment of those allergies should be pursued.

Naturopathic Manipulation

Naturopathy relies on natural remedies, such as sunlight, a healthy diet, and massage to treat illness. These concepts are certainly advisable to all patients to optimize the health of their entire mind and body and to minimize the effects of chronic pain. Herbal remedies are also often used. Some patients report success with these approaches but no formal studies have been conducted.

Osteopathic Manipulation

Osteopathy is a system of medicine based on the theory that disturbances in the musculoskeletal system affect other bodily parts. The thinking is that these disturbances cause many disorders. Likewise, the disorders can be corrected with various manipulative techniques in conjunction with conventional medical, surgical, pharmacological, and other therapeutic procedures.

Therapeutic Massage

Therapeutic massage involves the rubbing or kneading of body parts to improve circulation, relax the muscles, and provide sensory stimulation.

Physical Therapy (or Physiotherapy)

In this system, therapeutic exercises are used to treat physical dysfunction and injuries. Exercises are designed to restore normal functioning and development. Physical therapy may also include the application of heat, cold, vibration, ultrasound, biofeedback, or physical manipulation. This may help with muscle spasm and with nerve compression, both of which are adaptive responses to chronic pain. While physical therapy has been useful to some vulvodynia patients, the treatments all tend to vary. A standardized physical therapy protocol has not been published.

Traditional Chinese Medicine (Including Herbal Prescriptions and Acupuncture)

Traditional Chinese medical practices use medicinal herbs to prevent and treat diseases or ailments and also to promote health and healing. With acupuncture, specific body areas are pierced with fine needles to relieve pain. Some patients have reported success with Chinese medicinal practices. But all pain patients should exercise caution. Some herbal products on the market don't actually contain the herbs they claim to contain (and may even have chemicals or Western additives). Also, acupuncturists can sometimes be poorly trained and of variable skill. Research into the products you buy and people you trust is key.

Biofeedback

Biofeedback uses monitoring devices to furnish information regarding a bodily function, such as muscle tension or brainwaves, in an attempt to give the patient some voluntary control over that function. Biofeedback is used clinically to treat pain disorders by reducing stress reactions, rehabilitating muscles, and redirecting focused awareness.

Meditation and Stress Reduction Techniques

Meditation, hypnosis, and other states of self-regulation can help teach pain patients how to reduce their physiological and psychological states of arousal. Use of these techniques has been shown to reduce pain.

Yoga and Tai Chi

Yoga is an ancient discipline aimed at training the consciousness to achieve a state of perfect spiritual insight and tranquility. It incorporates a system of exercises to promote control of the body and mind. There are many styles of yoga—some such as Hatha yoga are more focused on physical postures; some focus more on the spiritual. There is a new trend in health clubs to offer "power yoga," a rapid series of yoga postures intended to give a cardiovascular workout. This form is less likely to be helpful for vulvar pain patients. Tai chi is a Chinese system of physical exercises designed especially for self-defense and meditation.

Both yoga and tai chi are ways of gently building strength and flexibility while helping you focus on the sensations of effective movement, and progressively improving overall function.

Family Therapy

This form of group psychotherapy involves treating one or more members of the family during the same session. Chronic pain causes changes in family dynamics; family therapy is useful for everyone involved.

Psychotherapy, Including Sexual Therapy

Psychotherapy encourages communication of conflicts and insight into problems in order to treat mental and emotional states. The goal is to relieve symptoms and change behavior to improve social and vocational functioning and increase personal growth. Sexual therapy can be especially helpful with vulvodynia patients. It is often conducted with couples and helps them maximize intimacy through loving, fulfilling sexual activity.

How to Make Chronic Pain Management Work for You

We know that you may still have a lot of questions. Here are some answers to questions often asked by people like you.

"How Do I Choose a Pain Management Facility?"

Pain management facilities will likely be under the supervision of anesthesiologists, neurologists, or psychiatrists. To find someone to help you:

1. Ask your doctor whether he knows of a pain specialist or clinic at his hospital or at a nearby major teaching hospital (affiliated with a medical school).

2. Once you choose a facility, call your insurance company to review your benefits. Ideally, you'll find a facility that is covered in your plan.

3. Call the chosen facility and ask to have the case manager speak to you about becoming a patient.

4. Interview the case manager and others about their experience with complicated pain and discuss any possible limitations or exclusions of your insurance and payment plans for services—specifically for patients with vulvodynia, interstitial cystitis, and other related disorders.

5. Ask about policy and procedures for patient rights and responsibilities, informed consent, billing procedures, and most importantly, for the credentials of practitioners.

"What Makes a Good Pain Management Professional?"

When you have located a doctor or facility that seems right for you, call your state medical licensing board to confirm they are licensed without restriction, and have not been involved in any prior disciplinary problems. (This is important as some pain management clinics have bad reputations.) In addition, your provider should have memberships in professional organizations at the state or national level. These organizations provide more opportunities for learning through continuing education courses. Finally, look for specialized training focused on pain issues, such as membership or diplomat status with the American Academy of Pain Management.

"Why Should I Bother to Find an Accredited Pain Program?"

Pain program accreditation speaks to several issues. First, it shows that these professionals are committed to the best possible organized care and the best treatments. Second, accreditation shows that your provider meets peer review standards for treating your problem. That is, the provider cares to compare his or her treatment outcomes to that of colleagues, and therefore devoted to constantly improving care and learning about the latest techniques. The bottom line is that accreditation means you get a program that has met the highest possible standards and has the patients' needs in mind.

"My Doctor Wants Me to Get Counseling—Is He Ditching Me?"

Absolutely not! Your physician just wants to be sure that you have comprehensive care. While pain is a physical issue, it affects all aspects of your life, including your mental health. A concerned doctor won't say your pain is in your head, but he or she will suggest that psychological techniques may help you deal with it more effectively. It's important to understand that pain causes stress and depression. This can be a vicious cycle. Psychotherapy can break the cycle and lead to more relief from your chronic pain. Also, some of the best medications for treating pain are drugs that are used for neurological and psychiatric therapy. Doctors who use these drugs for many patients may be good resources for helping adjust your regime to get the best results with the fewest side effects.

"How Can I Make Sure My Doctor Is Interacting with Me Properly?"

Here are some guidelines:

1. You should tell your doctor what your goals are at your first meeting. Your doctor should tell you what your treatment options are.

2. Your doctor should ask you for reports of your pain before, during, and after your courses of treatment.

3. You should have the chance to review your progress on a regular basis.

4. Your health care provider should ask you about your satisfaction with treatments.

5. You should feel like you're interacting and discussing your problem and treatments at every meeting.

"My Doctor Says There Is No Objective Basis for My Pain—Why?"

As you've read earlier, there may not be an explanation for why your chronic pain exists or any hard evidence that you're actually feeling pain. But that doesn't mean your pain isn't 100 percent real. Your doctor should take your subjective pain complaints quite seriously.

"Why Hasn't My Doctor Referred Me to a Pain Clinic Sooner?"

Conservative measures are usually tried before you are sent to a pain consultant. You may have persistent conditions that have not yet been brought under control, such as infections and dermatological disorders. However, if all known factors that could be causing your pain have been resolved, yet your pain has not resolved, it may be time for your doctor to refer you to a pain clinic.

"Are There Risks to Injections Used for Pain Management?"

There are potential risks any time the skin, a blood vessel, muscle, or nerve is injected. Most of the complications are minor and temporary. The treatment should be fully explained—including its adverse effects—prior to being performed. You should have the chance to ask questions and to sign a consent form.

"Is Pain Management Covered by Health Insurance?"

You always have to check with your specific provider. All policies are different. Check the benefits you qualify for.

Pain and the Workplace

Vulvodynia in the workplace is a complicated issue. Most sufferers are able to work—they juggle their pain and their job responsibilities well. But on occasion, women find themselves making multiple excuses for frequent doctor appointments, unpredictable side effects of medications, and other difficulties that stem from chronic pain. Most women may be tempted to tell their employers about their problem, but don't due to embarrassment or fear of the consequences.

Work environments can vary greatly, so whether or not to reveal your condition to your employer and coworkers is an important decision you have to make. Here are some suggestions from the National Vulvodynia Association on evaluating the pros and cons, and managing the condition while you're on the job.

1. Research your company's policies regarding disabilities, discrimination, and employment options such as flex time and telecommuting. Does your company have written polices on these issues? Are there minimum or maximum leave requirements? Job-sharing arrangements, for example, require a major commitment from both employer and employee.

   Deciding whether to tell your superiors is an important issue. Is your boss understanding? Do your supervisors seem tolerant of diversity? Consider how employees with other health problems have been treated to get an idea of what you can expect.

2. Why do you want to tell your boss? Do you want fewer responsibilities? Are you hoping to explain why your performance has been impaired or why you call in sick so often? Do you want to take a sick leave? If you want to change your hours, be sure you have a specific plan to propose.

3. Next, you must decide how much to tell. Do you want to tell your boss the whole story? For example, if you have vestibulitis and you're getting interferon injections, do you want to explain that? Some women just say that they have chronic gynecological pain. If you have a male boss, hearing that will usually stop him from asking more questions.

   If you are asking for a change in your work responsibilities, remember that your boss will have to tell his or her supervisor. Coworkers will want to know what is going on if you're not around as much anymore, especially if their workloads increase. You can tell them the truth, or you can just let them know you have a physical condition that interferes with your life and schedule. People may bombard you with concern and questions, so be prepared to have a response you're comfortable with. You don't have to tell anyone anything, but of course, you want to be polite. Remember that a decrease in your work may increase the work of others. They may be envious of your free time if they don't know the price you're paying to take it.

4. Keep in mind that, however unfair it may seem, the consequences of telling your employer about your condition could be negative. If you're up for a promotion, your boss may not think you can handle it. Or if you're already asking for a raise, this could affect whether you get it. Additionally, next time you change jobs, it may be more difficult to obtain health insurance with a pre-existing condition.

  One woman, a corporate manager, decided that telling her boss and taking a few days off every week were worth it. She could afford it financially, and she knew she needed more time to get better, rest, and function more successfully with her family. Other women may not feel the same way. However you decide to deal with this issue, it is your prerogative. You have the right and responsibility to do whatever works best for you. Just remember that your employer has a responsibility to his or her business and to other employees as well.

Your Employment Options

For more severe chronic sufferers, time off is the only suitable option. Some jobs involve sitting all day, which can be too difficult for vulvodynia patients. Others become so distracted by ongoing pain, or so affected by the medications they are taking, that they simply can't work. If either describes you, here are a few things to consider:

1. **Part-time Employment:** You'll have time for doctor's visits, therapies, and rest. You have to decide if you are willing to take a reduction in your salary until you get better. Be careful in making arrangements with the boss—some women complain that they end up working full-time for part-time pay.

2. **Job-sharing:** This can take two forms: Either two employees divvy up the work responsibilities and hours of one person, or they divide work according to their individual strengths. The benefits—and drawbacks—of job-sharing are similar to part-time work.

3. **Family and Medical Leave Act (FMLA):** In 1993, Congress passed this act, requiring companies with fifty or more employees to provide up to twelve weeks of unpaid leave during the calendar year for any of the following reasons: birth of or care for a child; placement of a child by adoption or foster care; care for a spouse, child, or parent if any have a serious health condition; a serious health condition which makes you unable to perform any of the essential functions of your position.

   Before taking your leave, make sure you'll be able to make the transition back to work when you're ready to come back. Check your insurance benefits while you're away as well. Taking a leave is an excellent way of evaluating if your job is affecting your health. It also gives you time to decide the next steps you want to take regarding work.

4. **Disability:** In extreme cases, disability may be appropriate. Policies vary with different employers, but in most cases you are eligible if you and your doctor declare that you are unable to perform the essential functions of your job due to a physical or mental impairment that substantially limits one or more of your life activities.

5. **Resigning:** If your company is inflexible, or you just can't take the daily routine of pain and work another second, you can offer to resign. Find out if there is a "force management program," or FMP. These are layoff plans that allow you to keep your retirement benefits, or at least part of them, and leave open the possibility of receiving your pension. This is a last-resort option that's worth looking into. Most women don't need to take such a drastic measure. In fact, it's best to keep working at a level that allows you to manage your pain and maintain your financial security and insurance benefits if you can. Often, the distractions of work, along with the financial, emotional, and intellectual rewards, can be helpful in keeping your mind off your pain. Work can also help ward off depression, which often accompanies chronic pain. Maybe your current situation is impossible. If so, and you decide to quit, it's beneficial to look for other creative outlets.

Chapter 7

Expressing Your Sexuality

Most women who suffer from vulvodynia experience pain with inter-course. As you know, your condition can have a devastating effect on your intimate relationships—even on your self-esteem. But know that you can reclaim your sexual identity.

One Sufferer's Sexual Ordeal

Jessica, twenty, has been dealing with the sexual issues of typical vulvodynia sufferers. Her story may hit close to home for many of you.

> *I started having sharp pain just outside the opening of my vagina shortly before I turned nineteen. Unfortunately, that happened right when I got married. At age twenty, I was formally diagnosed with vestibulitis. That first year, I had terrible problems with discomfort and pain. Here I was a newlywed, and I couldn't have sex. Sometimes I'd force myself and do it anyway. Of course, it was always horribly painful, and my husband couldn't understand. He thought he had somehow done something to me. Sometimes he'd think it was his fault; other times he would wonder what was wrong with me. It was so stressful on our relationship.*

After seeing three different doctors—I was in so much pain that I'd cry when they examined me—I was finally put on Elavil and told to refrain from sex. That wasn't difficult because I had no desire anyway. Penetration was torture, so why would I want any part of that? Within the next year, my husband and I couldn't take our personal and sexual problems anymore. We wound up divorced. It was awful for me at first. I felt completely alone and like everything that had happened was totally my fault. I thought something was so wrong with me and wondered if I was losing my mind. My family and closest friends couldn't help—they lived six hours away. Besides, I was too embarrassed to tell anyone about what I was going through. I worried about what people might think of me. It's no wonder I wound up really depressed.

In the last year, though, I've been feeling better. Slowly, the Elavil has helped. Plus, I joined a support group online and have received so much information and support from other women with the same problems. Finally, I had some hope.

Now I have an awesome, understanding boyfriend as well. He totally supports everything I do in trying to get better and holds my hand when I'm going crazy. I still don't have a very big sex drive because I'm always afraid it's going to hurt. But even that is slowly coming back. I have been able to have intercourse a few times without pain in the past year. That is because the vestibulitis is improving, my boyfriend is patient and understanding, and we go slowly using a lot of lubricant.

It was important to me to get back to having sex. For a while there, I felt like I had lost my sexual identity. I now know exactly how depressing and self-destructive that can be! I am seeing a new doctor now who encourages me and gives me tips for slowly going back to the sex life I enjoyed before vestibulitis. I finally realized that my boyfriend and I can enjoy sexual arousal and pleasure without intercourse. We don't feel as much pressure to "do the deed" anymore. If we can have intercourse, that's fine. But if we can't, we're both having wonderful physical intimacy (and orgasms!) without it.

*While sexual dysfunction isn't all there is to
vestibulitis, it had huge negative effects on my life. I'm so
much happier now that I am reconnecting with my sexual
self. Things are looking up for me.*

Vulvodynia and Sex

For women like Jessica, introital dyspareunia is a major component
in the diagnosis of vestibulitis.

As you've read in earlier chapters, the medical term for painful
intercourse is dyspareunia. There are two kinds—deep and superficial
(or introital). Deep, also called pelvic, dyspareunia is located further
back in the vagina and is present during thrusting. It is often related
to disorders such as uterine fibroids, endometriosis, and interstitial
cystitis. Typically, vulvar pain disorders do not cause deep
dyspareunia (although a woman can have vulvodynia and another
condition such as endometriosis at the same time).

On the other hand, superficial (also called introital) dyspareunia
is experienced at the opening of the vagina when the couple attempts
penetration. The pain is usually at the bottom of the vaginal opening
but can also occur all around that area. Dysesthetic vulvodynia patients
sometimes tolerate penetration a bit better because their pain is less
focused at the vestibule. For them, pain isn't just provoked by
sex—it's always there—but sexual activity can increase discomfort.

In summary, both vestibulitis and dysesthetic vulvodynia
patients report varying degrees of pain on initial insertion of the
penis, during thrusting, and after intercourse. In some cases,
vulvodynia pain is located higher up around the urethra, especially in
those women who experience frequent urinary tract symptoms. Pain
may also be located in the clitoris, though this is unusual. If the skin
is tight or there is a size difference between partners, the skin of the
fourchette may split, causing more pain.

Contributing Factors

Many factors contribute to dyspareunia. Some include infections,
vulvar skin disorders, hormone deficiencies, inadequate lubrication,
pelvic muscle tension, the penis size of the partner, lack of arousal,

and psychological states such as anxiety and depression. Health care providers should take a detailed and accurate sexual functioning history as part of the overall assessment of the vulvar pain condition. All too often, however, primary vulvar pain experts overlook the sufferer's sexuality. Gynecologists and dermatologists are often uncomfortable taking a detailed sexual history, and sadly, most are not trained to do so. Don't be put off if your ob/gyn just can't seem to solve your sexual problems. Seek out a well-trained professional who will talk to you and can help.

Also, remember not to beat yourself up over the inability to have sex. To put your situation in perspective, realize that most men will have erectile difficulties at some point in their lives. Before surgical procedures and, more recently, Viagra, many couples weren't able to complete intercourse due to male problems, which surely created relationship challenges. Many of these couples struggled to cope. Eventually, many also learned how to have fulfilling sex lives despite "equipment failure." For vulvar pain sufferers who have pain on touch or insertion, the situation is very similar. Keep in mind that human sexual functioning systems aren't perfect. Just like other parts of our bodies, our genitals can "get sick" and, luckily, can get better, too.

The Trap of Sexual Avoidance

Why is sexuality such a big deal in vulvar pain patients? Aren't there bigger problems—like pain—to deal with? Can't women and their partners live happy, healthy lives without sexual intimacy? And after all, won't most sufferers return to normal sexual activity after they're treated and their pain is reduced? The answer to all of the above is no, not usually. Once vulvodynia takes over, sex becomes an overwhelming obstacle for the women—and their partner(s). Studies prove what patients already know. Vulvodynia sufferers have far less sex than other women. One study reported that women ages twenty-five to twenty-nine have intercourse an average of seven and a half times every month (Laumann et al. 1994). By comparison, vestibulitis patients engage in sexual activity just four times a month (Binik and Bergeron 2001).

Let's take a closer look at what happens to the vast majority of vulvar pain sufferers with respect to their sexuality. Most women react by trying to have intercourse, despite their problems with it. They don't want to disappoint their partners or turn away the one they love. While well-intentioned, this common practice is not a good idea. Why? Because the woman naturally begins to associate sexual activity with pain. Next thing she knows, any time she thinks of sexual arousal, pleasure, intimacy, and intercourse, she has a negative knee-jerk reaction. Her desire then sharply decreases.

Many sufferers report this loss of libido. When asked about their sexual activity, vulvar pain patients frequently say they don't want to talk about it. "At this point, sex is the last thing in the world that interests me," is a common report.

Our bodies help us remain emotionally and behaviorally functional when we're faced with pain. How? By automatically defocusing or distracting our awareness away from the sources of the pain. Sex is a source of pain, so sufferers concoct elaborate plans to avoid it at all costs. Even more basically, though, the vulva is a source of pain, so patients try not to think about it. While this is quite functional for everyday living and avoidance of discomfort, it obviously creates a huge problem. Your body part that is producing pain—namely your vulva—becomes a pariah. Yet it is still a part of you! This is why so many women also suffer from anxiety and depression, loss of self-esteem and loss of sexual identity.

Sufferers begin to change all aspects of their lives to avoid the possibility of physical intimacy. They do this both unconsciously and consciously. For example, some women start going to bed earlier or later than their partners. Or they purposely become too busy at work or home—with the sole purpose of avoiding sexual encounters. One patient even revealed to us that she stopped going to romantic movies because the sex scenes triggered her own feelings of anxiety, depression, and inadequacy. She couldn't stand to be reminded that she had no sex life of her own.

How Sex Benefits Your Life

Sexuality is not just designed for pleasure. By avoiding it, you miss out on its many health benefits. Getting back to sex is more important than you think. Here's why:

1. Sex reduces pain. It's a medical fact: The more sexually aroused you are, the more pain your body can tolerate. If you

and your partner can reach high levels of excitement, your pain is more likely to subside, which will allow you to enjoy yourself. (Bonus for vulvodynia sufferers: High arousal means your partner will reach orgasm faster. This can be a blessing for you if you can tolerate only brief sexual activity.)

2. Frequent sexual activity keeps genital tissue healthier. Arousal causes the pelvic region to circulate with blood, which rebuilds and refuels cells, muscles, glands, and vulvar skin. Using your sexual body parts also keeps them "tuned up" and keeps them strong and fit.

3. Sex keeps couples intimately and happily connected. Sexual encounters mean shared vulnerability for partners. This is the willingness to expose our less-than-perfect selves. You do not expose yourself in this way to just anyone—only to the person you love and trust the most. Being intimate with this person strengthens your ties to one another. In pleasing your partner (and vice versa), you'll keep the door open to a rewarding sex life even if you continue to have limitations on some activities (such as intercourse).

Partner Problems

You can see how avoidance of intercourse can cause problems for you. It can also be a problem for your partner—and your relationship. Katherine, forty-eight, writes:

I am fortunate to have an understanding fiancée—we've been together since before I was diagnosed with dysesthetic vulvodynia. However, as supportive as he is, it is disappointing for him (and for me!) because our first year together was full of sexual intercourse. It's been very difficult for him to go without it. While I sympathize, it's hard for me. I'm the one in pain! This situation is incredibly difficult for both of us and has resulted in a lot of hurt and disagreement in our relationship.

As you probably know, partners are greatly affected by vulvodynia, too. Whether it is a straight or gay relationship, the effects on the significant other are the same. First of all, the healthy partner loathes watching the vulvodynia sufferer deal with pain and unpleasantness. It's frustrating and sad. No one wants to see a loved one suffer. And he or she probably feels exasperated because there's nothing to do that will help. He (we'll refer to the sufferer's partner in the male form from now on simply to avoid confusion) then realizes that his partner with vulvodynia is only agreeing to have sex to fulfill his needs. That becomes unfulfilling for him—and even worrisome. For as much as he wants to have sex with his partner, he certainly doesn't enjoy knowing that he's hurting her. As you can see, the whole idea of sexual activity becomes complicated extremely quickly. In fact, many men report loss of arousal and difficulty in maintaining erections. The sufferer's sexual dysfunction results in his own sexual dysfunction.

Simple Miscommunication

Classic miscommunication occurs on several levels. In the realm of physical contact, each partner wants to feel he or she is giving what the other person wants. The woman sufferer tries to have sex to please her significant other. Her partner refrains because he knows the woman experiences pain with sex. Neither person will be happy. The issues become more complicated as time goes on. And as sufferers know all too well, vulvodynia can be a long-lasting, recurrent problem.

Miscommunication, of course, goes even deeper than misunderstandings about sex. A lot of times in heterosexual relationships, men just aren't going to express their feelings about vulvodynia as much as women do. Some men may not show the sufferer the attention or understanding that she expects. Many of the most well-meaning males simply don't know how to show their sympathetic sides. (They are not brought up to express their sweet, mushy sides. In fact, they often try to hide highly emotional feelings.) Another possibility: The male may be avoiding intimate discussion because he assumes that a heart-to-heart will lead to another less than satisfying attempt at intercourse, with pain for her and guilt for him. It may seem uncaring to gripe about his desire for pleasure in the context of her chronic pain.

Anger

Anger is a normal feeling for couples who are dealing with a chronic, dehabilitating condition. It doesn't matter which partner is suffering! For vulvodynia patients, in particular, it usually goes like this:

You're angry because no one seems to help or understand you. At different times, you may feel shunned by doctors, employers, and even loved ones. You may feel like your partner has no idea what you go though. If he wants to have sex, and you're having a painful day, you may feel anger. Meanwhile, he may be angry because he feels rejected. He wants to be supportive and understanding, but he also wants to maintain a loving, intimate relationship with the woman he loves.

The way to handle anger is to simply be aware of it. Know that it exists (especially on already stressful days), and that feeling it is normal and healthy. Just put it in its place and don't let it last long. Whenever tension is down, couples need to reassure each other that they're trying to be understanding and caring. Bouts of anger sting less when couples remind one another of their love and commitment. You may not be able to take away the cause of the anger, but you might be able to do things to make your partner happy in other ways that don't have anything to do with sex. Sometimes just seeing your commitment to his happiness can strengthen his commitment to your comfort. So just ask him, "Is there anything I can do to make your day better?"

Reconnection

Chronic pain can throw couples off-kilter over and over again. But couples are far more likely to bounce back from challenges (and lack of sex is a big challenge!) if they maintain their love and connection. Sexually speaking, it's important that couples remind each other they are intimate partners regardless of what is—or isn't—going on in the bedroom. After all, without sexual connection, couples are more like close friends or roommates. While various forms of sexual play may not be possible, other intimate gestures are. Try playing touching games when you're alone. For example, if you pinch his behind or tickle his shoulder, you're telling him that you like his body in a light, fun, humorous way. (This works the other way around, of course.) Anyway couples reassure each other sexually, even without sexual activity, will help strengthen their connection.

Another way to strengthen your relationship is to initiate acceptable sexual activity. Even if you're not able to have penetration, showing interest in sex tells him you still find him sexy and appealing. Plus, if you, the sufferer, show sexual interest, you take a lot of pressure off of your partner. He may be scared to initiate activity because he doesn't want to hurt you. But he will welcome it when you show interest first, and guide him to what activity *is* pleasurable and desired.

Finding a Mate

If you are not in a relationship, you may find that meeting someone is a lot harder because you have vulvodynia. Here's a typical story from a young woman named Sarah:

> *I'm an attractive, successful twenty-six-year-old woman in New York City. I am a party planner, so I meet hot eligible men nearly every day. It's happened to me over and over. I will meet a guy I have a lot in common with, and we go out several times. Things go along smoothly, and we really seem to click. But the relationship stagnates because I can't take it to higher sexual levels. I have been suffering from vestibulitis for four years and penetration is nearly impossible. When I tell this to the guys I date, they try to act understanding, but I can tell they're skeptical. They think I'm a psychological mess; that I make everything up to avoid sex, or that I'm just a plain, old prude. I have never felt like they really understand what my pain feels like or what I go through both emotionally and physically. It's especially frustrating for me because in my early twenties I loved sex. I had amazing, memorable sexual interludes with several different partners.*
>
> *So, no matter how great I get along or connect with guys now, I can't seem to keep a boyfriend longer than two months. I am sure it's because I can't have sex. It's terribly*

sad for me. I want to find someone special and get married one day. I'd even like to have children. I am afraid I will wind up alone.

Dating is much more difficult for single women who are unable to have intercourse. Many sufferers already have partners when their vulvodynia symptoms begin. They are able to enjoy sex for a period of time before they start having problems with intercourse. For all of their relationship difficulties, at least they have memories of sex—and a loving, established relationship—to fall back on.

What about women who suffer alone? While they might have opportunities to go out with men, like Sarah, they worry that nothing will last because of their inability to have sex. Some avoid dating all together because a) they don't want to fall for someone who will dump them over sex, or b) they don't want to suffer the embarrassment of telling potential partners that they can't consummate the relationship.

These women often wind up feeling like slaves to their vulvodynia. But there is hope for them. First and foremost, these women desperately need to find good treatment from excellent professionals. The truth is that most vulvodynia sufferers who seek the care of vulvar pain specialists experience significant levels of relief. Most of them are able to return to various levels of sexual activity.

But even then, some single women suffer emotional consequences—especially if they've been rejected in the past due to their vulvodynia. If you are single and recovering from vulvodynia, you may benefit from psychological counseling.

During treatment, even if pain is still persistent, single women should try to date if they so desire. Mature partners who are able to handle vulvodynia physically and emotionally do exist. One woman, Tara, age twenty-five, found a great guy. She and her now-husband dated two years before getting married. On their second wedding anniversary, they still had *never* had sexual intercourse. It was simply too painful for her each time she tried. The couple didn't try again until her treatments began to work and her pain subsided. With sexual counseling, Tara and her partner are now enjoying a satisfying sex life.

The above scenario is possible for other singles. They have to do three things while dating: pursue effective treatment for their problem; find a sympathetic partner; and keep up some level of sexual activity. That is exactly what Tara did. For the four years she and her partner were unable to have intercourse, they tried every other sexual activity in the book—and enjoyed it. They did not let the lack of intercourse affect their ability to enjoy pleasure together.

Single women can certainly give pleasure—the problem for them is that they have reservations about receiving it, mainly due to concerns about pain. Singles should focus more on non-intercourse sexual activities that they enjoy, alone and with partners. Just because you're single and suffer from vulvodynia doesn't mean you should go without sexual pleasure.

How to Enjoy Sex Again

The sexual tensions that arise as a result of vulvodynia should not stop patients and their partners from all attempts at intercourse. It can be helpful for patients to progressively maintain intercourse attempts but to always stop when the pain becomes significant. Here's how to do this most successfully. *After sufficient sexual arousal that includes adequate vaginal lubrication*, try to have intercourse by putting the head of the penis (or if the couple prefers, a penis-like pleasuring device) at the opening of the vagina. Then the couple should move very slowly and gently toward deeper insertion. Start by placing the head inside the vagina and moving forward from there.

Remember, it's important to stop attempting penetration the second that significant pain occurs. At this point other sexually plea-surable techniques (see descriptions and how-tos below) should be employed. Still, the gentle insertion method helps the sufferer get valuable information about the state of her pain and effectiveness of her courses of treatment. Most importantly, she won't associate vagi-nal penetration with pain. Instead, sexual activity can still remain pleasurable for both people.

Intercourse Isn't Everything

If a simple gentle penetration technique were the complete answer to couples' issues of sexuality, the problem could be easily solved. But as most of you know, there's a lot more to it. Unfortu-nately for most sufferers, the pain experienced with intercourse is only the beginning. First of all, most women—those who didn't try the gentle penetration technique as soon as they began having vulvar pain—have already had extremely uncomfortable intercourse. And they've probably had it many times, meaning they've already developed negative attitudes about sex. They've already experienced the frustration, shame, and embarrassment of having too much pain to engage in intercourse.

So it's no surprise that they have already started avoiding intercourse all together.

That brings us to the next point. Unfortunately, for the vast majority of people, sex *is* intercourse. How often do you hear people use the word *sex* as if it were synonymous with intercourse? All other forms of non-penetrative sexual activity are relegated to the realm of foreplay, which by definition refers to what people do to get ready for intercourse. With this common line of thinking, afflicted couples avoid "starting what they can't finish," as it were. This is a huge mistake.

Sufferers and their partners need to realize that while intercourse isn't always possible, other forms of physical, sexual, and pleasurable intimacy are. Please don't fall into the trap of avoiding all kinds of physical closeness. Keep in mind that even if intercourse hurts, something else that's sexual *must* feel good. Have a certain spot that makes you purr? Make sure it's stimulated! Find out what turns you on, and focus your sexual attention in that area. Ask your partner to become involved. Then work on making that certain something a regular part of your life that you look forward to.

Interestingly, surveys show that people privately value several different kinds of non-intercourse sexual activity (Klein and Robbins 1998). Although they don't admit it readily, men and women alike enjoy masturbation, sensual massage, oral sex, anal sex, and manual stimulation. Yet intercourse is ingrained as the "norm." Getting away from the idea that intercourse is the only acceptable option is key for sufferers seeking to reclaim sexual pleasure.

Non-Intercourse Sex Activities

Not sure which non-intercourse activities to try? Look through women's magazines for articles with titles like "25 Ways to Make Him Moan." Surprisingly, the sex tips in those articles often include non-penetrative, fun, and easy sexual stunts. We've also included a few ideas below. You can try them alone or with a partner. Many are adapted from Marty Klein's book, *Let Me Count the Ways* (1998).

1. Be sensual. Reestablish your sensual self. Listen to music that makes you feel sexy. Buy your favorite lotion and put it on slowly after a relaxing bath. Treat yourself to nice lingerie that makes you feel good about your body. Read stories or books that stimulate sexual thoughts and desire (like romance novels or the racy works of author Nancy Friday). Go on romantic, intimate dates to quiet restaurants. And try to talk to your partner about the things—big and small—that turn you on. (Even if they're outrageous or silly!)

2. Kiss. Whether romantic smooches are on television, in the movies, or in real life, they offer powerful connections for couples.

3. Masturbate alone. Enough said. Don't be afraid to engage in this self-loving activity.

4. Masturbate together. This activity can be done several ways. It's especially useful for each person to masturbate him- or herself while the partner watches. (Then the partner can see *exactly* what kind of touches and moves will work!) Couples can masturbate themselves at the same time, so they experience sexual pleasure together.

5. Engage in oral sex. Many men and women report that oral sex produces more orgasms than intercourse, mutual masturbation, and just about any other bedroom activity. By stimulating someone's genitals with the mouth, the giver is showing total acceptance of the partner. They are also supplying extreme pleasure. Helpful hint: Don't rush oral sex, and don't try to do it perfectly. Whether you're giving or receiving it, take time to enjoy every moment of sensation and intimacy.

6. Focus on nipple stimulation. With fingers, mouth, teeth, vibrating objects, and different temperatures, you can pull, twist, pinch, nibble, lick, suck, tease, and taste each other's nipples. Experiment a lot with this to see what feels good

for each partner. While rare, some women can even have orgasms from the perfect nipple stimulation.

7. Look at each other. No matter what kind of sexual activity you and your partner are enjoying, remember to make eye contact and talk. Some experts believe that making these important connections during sex helps lovers tolerate more intense pleasure and pain.

8. Practice massage. Use oils, fragrances, fingers, feathers, or whatever else strikes your fancy, to caress each other's bodies. A variety of kneading, light, and intense touch should be used. Remember that touch is more pleasurable when it is unexpected. So during massage, keep each other guessing.

9. Be an exhibitionist. Show off your body to your partner. Cook dinner naked, go without underwear, or grope your partner under a table in a public restaurant. "Accidentally" flash each other sexy patches of flesh.

10. Talk sexy. Whisper naughty nothings into each other's ear before sexual play to get in the mood. Try having steamy conversations over the phone, before you see each other in the evening. Tell your partner what you'd like to do to him, and what he could do to you. Also, you can use sexy sentences during sexual activity to further arouse your partner. (Hint: Compliment each other's bodies, techniques, and anatomy often.)

11. Play with food. Put a few simple snacks such as fruit, candy, ice cream, or whipped cream on your partner's body. Slowly lick it off, relishing the taste slowly and carefully.

12. Employ sex toys. If you and your partner have never brought sex items into the bedroom, this is an option to consider. Many "toys" don't require vaginal insertion. But they do vibrate on various body parts, especially the clitoris. Vibrators, available online from various retailers, are especially helpful to get vulvodynia sufferers back to enjoying sex. Hint: Most women, even those without pain, prefer not to have direct contact of the vibrator on the clitoris. At first,

try applying it nearby or over your fingers to soften the sensation. (This is even more importnat if you have dysesthesia). Experimenting with different products—for men and women—can add a new satisfying dimension to intercourse-free sexual activity.

Finding Professional Help to Heal Your Sexual Issues

Despite problems such as the loss of desire, the inability to have intercourse, and a general disinterest in all sexual activity, most vulvar pain sufferers cling desperately to the belief that when their vulvar pain is eliminated or significantly reduced, they will just return to their previous, normal level of sexual activity. Unfortunately, this is just not what happens. After years of treating and counseling patients, we have found that it takes more work than that.

Since both sexual and psychological matters tend to bring up a great deal of resistance and embarrassment, very often physicians inadvertently conspire with you to avoid discussing these matters. The physicians themselves prefer to stick to dealing with infections and tissue, which is what they are trained to do, and often avoid confronting the sufferer on the sexual and psychological consequences of their vulvar pain. In one study (Glazer 2000), several follow-ups were done with patients who said they were completely pain-free after completing their treatments. Three to five years after having no vulvar pain, these women reported that their sex lives had not returned to their pre-vulvodynia levels. Their sex lives had not improved the way they had hoped—their levels of sexual interest, the frequency of sex, and the experience of sexual pleasure just hadn't returned to their former states. This is yet another example of how important it is to integrate vulvodynia treatment with sex therapy. Doctors, psychologists, and other professionals need to be involved with your progress every step of the way. That is the only way the health care community can hope to restore patients to their previous levels of psychological well-being and sexual functioning.

Beware of Bad Sexual Advice

Unfortunately, some professionals may still hold negative attitudes about sex that won't help you. Well-meaning friends and family can sometimes give you destructive messages about your sexuality. Below, look at the mistaken ideas many people have about sex (Klein and Robbins 1998). Avoid seeking help and advice from those who send you these emphatically false messages:

1. Any sexual problems you have are all in your head.

2. Sex really shouldn't worry anyone all that much. Instead, be grateful for all of the other things you have.

3. Sex is not that important to our lives anyway.

4. Instead of constantly thinking about your sexual dysfunction, concentrate on being more normal in other areas of your life.

5. Sex will be better if you can convince your partner to change.

6. Just give up sex completely; it may not be for you.

7. Get it through your head that men and women are just sexually incompatible.

8. Your sexual situation may improve if you find a new partner (or have an affair).

9. Use your sexuality to manipulate your partner. Use techniques such as teasing, flaunting, withholding, and threatening to get what you want.

A Treatment That Works

Psychosexual issues about vulvar pain should be addressed right from the beginning. This ultimately leads to a much more satisfactory outcome for the patient. We even encourage our patients who are in relationships to bring their significant others to the office with them for their initial evaluation. With the permission of the patient, we invite the partner to participate in the evaluation and together we address both relationship and sexual issues. Those patients who are not in relationships, or those who prefer not to have their partner participate, we see individually for detailed psychosexual evaluations.

We frankly discuss issues of sexual conduct, including intercourse, oral/manual stimulation, and masturbation. We frequently find that patient shyness and/or lack of sexual knowledge significantly limits the sufferer's ability to experience their sexual thoughts and experiences. We are also careful to respect the moral, religious, or personal boundaries set by the patient.

But we do encourage them to open up. Why? Because as a recent study shows, the use of sexual therapy in addition to other treatments vastly improves sexual functioning in vulvar vestibulitis patients (Bergeron et al. 2001).

How We Incorporate Sexuality

We work with sufferers either individually or as a couple and begin the resexualization process as early as possible. We work to help patients recapture not only sexual activity but also their sexual identities as women and as loving partners. We start with cognitive restructuring, which helps women to view themselves and their sexuality in a positive light—even as they continue to experience limitations on their sexual conduct. Slowly, sexual activity is restarted, usually with masturbation exercises. This helps patients reexperience, or in some cases experience for the first time, orgasm through self-stimulation. Focus is put on a fulfilling sexual experience, not just on the mechanical performance of the sexual activity. Patients are encouraged to reconnect with their rich sexual fantasy lives and to explore all forms of self-stimulation, which works to enhance arousal.

We also teach various forms of relaxation. This helps patients stop associating sexual arousal with pain. Patients must understand that arousal is not purely a sexual activity, but also promotes physiological health in the vulva and vagina. Sexual arousal mechanisms in the female genitals rely heavily on vasocongestion—that is, when the genitals fill up with blood (much like when the penis fills with blood in males and causes an erection). Increased blood flow to the area is good for the tissue—and many patients do not have good blood circulation in their pelvic region. Also, good blood flow is essential for experiencing an orgasm. Further, orgasms are greatly beneficial to the pelvic floor musculature. Climaxing can help in restoring vulvodynia patients' abnormal, tense, spastic pelvic muscles. (The physiology underlying an orgasm is actually the just-under-a-second rhythmic contractions of the fast-twitch fiber of the pubococcygeus muscle, and therefore orgasms can be beneficial for the health of the pelvic floor musculature.)

With these resexualizing techniques, many of our patients begin to return to their previous levels of sexual functioning. They also experience a welcomed, renewed interest in physical intimacy. These activities also help our patients learn more about their own bodies, such as how to best stimulate their genital area, and how best to achieve states of maximum sexual arousal. While the first steps in resexualization are underway, we also work with patients to improve communication with their partners before focusing on partner sex. Partner sex is then started with a focus on mutual non-penetrative stimulation, i.e., oral and manual sex.

In cases where tightness of the vulvar skin or hymen are a problem, or when penis size is an issue, we introduce the use of dilators, penis-like devices that help to stretch the vaginal opening, and self/partner finger insertion. This prepares the tissue for future comfortable penile insertion. Of course, the specific progression of sexual activity depends on the individual patient, and her specific goals.

We make sexual rehabilitation an important part of the overall treatment. We strongly believe multidisciplinary integrative treatment is necessary to fully restore our patients to health—and we hope other facilities across the nation do, too.

When looking for help with sexual issues, you may ask friends, family, even professionals for help. Of course, it's best to seek out a whole-self approach to treatment. But depending on where you live and your resources (including insurance benefits), you may not have access to total-care vulvar pain therapy. If that's the case, go to an ob/gyn and sex therapist separately, asking if they can coordinate with each other on your progress. Make sure you are receiving caring advice that you feel good about.

Pregnancy for Sufferers

Coauthor Gae Rodke is not only a vulvar pain specialist, but she also delivers babies. Many vulvar pain specialists don't do both. Since the bulk of her patients are vulvodynia sufferers, she has unique experience with pain symptoms and pregnancy. She provides information for mothers-to-be below.

Getting Pregnant

Vulvar pain is not associated with infertility, as Howard Glazer's survey shows. While that is a fortunate truth, it doesn't make getting pregnant (i.e., having intercourse) any easier. For some women, there are times when sexual intercourse is virtually impossible. So what should a woman of childbearing years do?

She should go ahead and try. If everything else is normal—her periods, his sperm count—calculating the fertile period is simple. Subtract fourteen from the average length of the menstrual cycle to find the probable day of ovulation. Two to three days before that are your most fertile days. For example, in a thirty-day cycle with day one as the first day of menses, meaning bleeding, the two to three days prior to day sixteen would be the best time to get pregnant. (Sometimes you can tell where you are in your cycle by closely inspecting your discharge. Often, a clear mucus discharge—as opposed to the milkier discharge that occurs later in the cycle—is a sign of ovulation.) As for the sperm, they seem to work most effectively when they're already in the area when the egg comes along, which is why you need to have sex before ovulation. The sperm must pass through the cervix into the uterus, then it must travel up the fallopian tubes, and be ready and waiting when ovulation occurs. Having intercourse the day of or after ovulation is less likely to produce a pregnancy.

Trying to Get Pregnant

That said, since vulvodynia patients often have bouts of unpredictable dyspareunia, actually having sex is another issue. Topical Xylocaine solution can be applied to the vaginal opening with a cotton ball. Tuck the cotton ball into the space between the labia minora just outside the hymen for ten minutes prior to attempted penetration. Then place it right at the opening prior to intercourse to numb the area. Be careful not to get the medicine on the penis, or he'll be numbed too, and getting to ejaculation will take longer. Also be sure to keep the Xylocaine away from the clitoris—an area you don't want to be numbed!

For women with pain on insertion, longer isn't usually better. You should also use lubricants. A good one is Astroglide, which is available at the drug store. Naturally occurring oils such as vegetable oils (yes, the kind you cook with) are also good lubricants and easily available, or look for a water-based solution that has the fewest preservatives. Avoid petroleum-based lubricants or anything with perfumes in it. Why use lubrication if the area is numbed? To decrease friction and reduce irritation after the anesthetic wears off. A cold compress afterward also helps minimize irritation later.

Of course, some patients can be inseminated in the doctor's office if they absolutely can't have intercourse, but that is rarely the case. Some couples resort to at-home methods. "One couple in my practice used a turkey baster to insert the husband's sperm into the wife's vagina," wrote Stanley Marinoff, M.D. "And the result was twins" (1996). Or try placing semen into a new diaphragm (never used with spermicide) and then placing it directly over the cervix.

Gynecological exams and procedures may be more uncomfortable for patients with vulvar pain. Exams during labor and manipulation to accomplish delivery may also cause discomfort, which can be relieved by "regional" anesthesia, such as epidural. Postpartum hormonal changes and tender scars can increase vulvar pain. While none of the above are fun, they are usually tolerable and often treatable. Fortunately, the fetus is rarely affected by the pain or these treatments. Overall, pain usually remains the same as before the pregnancy; rarely is it worse except in the immediate postpartum period. Occasionally it is even improved. There is also no evidence that a cesarean section produces a better outcome, in terms of vulvar pain, than a vaginal delivery.

Pregnancy and Medication

The fetus may be affected by medications the mother takes to manage pain. Patients taking tricyclic antidepressants, anticonvulsants, and other oral meds should try to wean themselves off or switch to medications with longer records of safety. There are no direct studies on these drugs' effects on the fetus, so don't take chances unnecessarily. The first trimester, when the fetus is being formed, is the most important time to avoid taking meds. If you're trying to get pregnant or suspect that you are, early detection is key. The earlier you stop, the better. Of course, sometimes a patient can't tolerate complete discontinuation—if you're in that situation, ask your doctor if he'll consider giving you a lower dose or a different medicine while you're pregnant.

It's been found that amitriptyline, a commonly used tricyclic antidepressant, does cross into the placenta and is excreted in breast milk. Animal studies of the impact of amitriptyline and nortriptyline on the fetus have yielded inconclusive results. Use of antihistamines, such as hydroxyzine, is less problematic, but should be monitored by a doctor. Patients using topical steroid medications may be advised to decrease the potency or frequency of use. Also, patients should minimize the use of topical testosterone while trying to conceive, and after a positive pregnancy test, they should be switched to progesterone promptly (Rodke 2000).

Patients using biofeedback for pain management should keep doing so because it actually improves the muscles before and after delivery. Following the low-oxalate diet is safe, as long as a physician monitors it to make sure the mother receives all of the vitamins and nutrients she needs. Also, calcium citrate—about 1200 to 1500 milligrams per day—is safe to take while pregnant (Marinoff 1996).

Pregnancy and Pain

Most patients don't have more pain during pregnancy than they had before. Some patients even improve. One exception: Women with chronic yeast infections may find that their symptoms get worse. Pregnancy makes the vagina warmer and more moist, which increases the growth of candidal organisms. Chronic skin conditions, such as lichen sclerosus, are often improved, probably due to increased levels of progesterone made by the placenta.

Treating yeast infections during pregnancy is a bit different. It's important for the physician to distinguish between Candida albicans and the non-albicans varieties. During the first trimester, internal treatment should be withheld unless absolutely necessary. External treatment during this time can give symptomatic relief with safe, older medications such as nystatin (for albicans and non-albicans) or miconazole (for albicans). Diflucan and Ancobon, modern yeast treatments, should be avoided during attempts at conception and during pregnancy because they are absorbed systemically (Rodke 2000).

Pre-Delivery

Fortunately, vulvodynia patients don't require cesarean deliveries any more than other patients, even if they've had a vestibulectomy. Vulvodynia alone is certainly no cause for a cesarean section. Of course, as in any pregnancy, other reasons may arise for cesarean delivery. However, in my experience, as well as that of Dr. Marinoff, most women with vulvodynia deliver successfully via the vagina.

Once in labor, a newer "walking" epidural anesthetic is preferable to the older kind. This gives pain relief without loss of muscle power for the first two to four hours. Afterward, a continuous infusion of local anesthetic through the epidural catheter keeps the woman comfortable. The rate of infusion can be adjusted and reduced slightly during pushing to allow a better sense of timing and for direction of the pushing effort. The "walking" epidural also makes it easier to control the rate of delivery. By removing pain and the overwhelming urge to get the baby out as quickly as possible, the doctor or midwife can coach the patient to push steadily with greater or lesser effort to ease the baby out with the least possible trauma. The goal of the medical care provider should be to avoid creating tears and scars in an already painful area, which is, of course, the vestibule and perineum.

Vulvodynia sufferers should definitely seek out an obstetrician or certified nurse midwife who is experienced with and cares about "intact delivery." Episiotomy or lacerations, cuts, or tears in the perineal tissue at the base of the vaginal opening should be avoided especially in vulvodynia and lichen sclerosus patients (Rodke 2000). Why? A new scar in that area will result in a new focus of tenderness. An episiotomy can make vulvodynia worse. The exception would be in cases of emergency, when a few extra minutes to allow delivery without trauma is not in the best interest of the fetus. In fact, episiotomies should be avoided in almost all deliveries, according to more recent research. Incisions are almost always larger than they would be if the woman tore naturally. Incisions are also more likely to cause damage to the rectal sphincter and the rectum.

Finding a physician or midwife who is dedicated to delivering without episiotomy can be a challenge. Delivery without episiotomy is not simply a matter of allowing spontaneous uncontrolled birth; it is an active collaborative process between the woman and her attendant. Once the baby's head is crowning, the mother should pant or blow instead of pushing during the next few contractions. This allows the tissues to stretch without tearing. Unmedicated patients will feel the sensation of burning as the tissues stretch. When that happens, blow, don't push.

Some practitioners recommend perineal massage to prepare the vulvar tissue for delivery. Studies have shown variable results (Klein and Robbins 1998). Many vulvar pain patients, especially those who experience pain on touch, find perineal massage uncomfortable. It isn't necessary if a woman can't handle it. The advantages are not sufficient to justify the pain massaging may cause (Rodke 2000).

Post-Delivery

Most women (vulvodynia sufferers or not!) experience some discomfort and frustration during the postpartum phase. In addition to possible vulvar/vaginal trauma, the decrease in vaginal estrogenization that occurs with lactation can cause dryness and burning. Small amounts of estrogen cream may be helpful. Vaginal lubricants may also ease symptoms. It is unusual for permanent increases in vulvar pain to occur. The stretching of the introital skin may be beneficial in reducing the friction once sexual intercourse resumes. Also, if pelvic floor exercises are performed correctly, the vaginal muscular tone can be improved, causing a vast improvement in function and comfort (Rodke 2000).

Most medications appear in breast milk, some in greater concentration than others. Some have been used safely by breastfeeding moms for conditions such as depression. The mother should discuss the pluses and minuses of drug therapy and breastfeeding with her doctor.

Vulvodynia can be a great challenge. As you've learned from the information in this book, caring compassionate treatment and realistic positive expectations can help you adequately manage and enjoy a fulfilling life. We wish you all the best in your journey toward healing.

Appendix A

Glossary

Acute: A condition of sudden onset and short duration. The opposite of acute is chronic. A chronic condition is long-lasting.

Allergy: A rapid response from the body's immune system against a foreign substance. Allergy symptoms can range from a runny nose and nasal congestion to hives. In its most severe form, called "anaphylaxis," it may be associated with a significant drop in blood pressure, closing down of the breathing passages, and even death.

Allodynia: The experience of pain in response to a stimulus which should produce a normal sensation of touch. The sensation of pinching, cutting, or scraping in the vulva caused by the light touch of a cotton swab is vulvar allodynia.

Amitriptyline: A tricyclic andidepressant used in low doses to treat chronic pain. Other medications in this class include nortriptyline, desipramine, doxepin, and imipramine.

Anesthetic: Medications that decrease the sensation of pain. A topical anesthetic is applied directly to a surface. Lidocaine and EMLA are examples of topical anesthetics frequently used to treat vulvar pain.

Antibiotics: Medications commonly used to treat bacterial infections. Most antibiotics are not effective against fungal or viral infections.

Anticholinergic medications: These medications cause relaxation of the muscles within the bladder, and may also affect the muscle within the intestines, sometimes causing constipation. They are also well-known to cause dryness of the mouth because of their ability to decrease saliva production. Tricyclic antidepressants, such as amitriptyline, often used to treat vulvar pain, can have significant anticholinergic side effects.

Anticonvulsants: Originally developed for the treatment of seizures, these medications have been found to be effective in the treatment of chronic pain disorders, including vulvar pain. They include carbamazepine (Tegretol), Dilantin, and most recently, gabapentin (Neurontin).

Asymptomatic: Having no symptoms.

Atrophic vaginitis: A condition in which the lining of the vagina loses thickness and becomes thin and dry. This usually is caused by a loss of estrogen and can result in symptoms of vaginal itching and/or burning, loss of vaginal lubrication, and discomfort with sexual intercourse.

Autoimmune diseases: Illnesses that occur when the body tissues are attacked by its own immune system, a complex organization within the body that is designed normally to "seek and destroy" invaders of the body, particularly infections. Patients with these diseases frequently have unusual antibodies in their blood that target their own body tissues. Examples of autoimmune diseases include systemic lupus erythematosus, Sjogren's syndrome, Hashimoto's thyroiditis, rheumatoid arthritis, and juvenile diabetes mellitus. Autoimmune diseases are more common in women than in men. Furthermore, the presence of one autoimmune disease increases your chances for developing another simultaneous autoimmune disease.

Biofeedback: The technique of making unconscious or involuntary bodily processes (such as the activity of your pelvic floor muscles) perceptible (often through demonstration on a computer screen) so that you can manipulate them by conscious mental control.

Biological response modifiers (BRMs): Substances that stimulate the body's response to infection and disease. The body naturally produces small amounts of these substances, and scientists can produce some of them in the laboratory in large amounts for use in treating cancer, rheumatoid arthritis, and other diseases. BRMs used in biological therapy include monoclonal antibodies, interferon, interleukin-2 (IL-2), and several types of colony-stimulating factors (CSF, GM-CSF, G-CSF). Interleukin-2 and interferon are BRMs being tested for the treatment of advanced malignant melanoma. Interferon is already used to treat hepatitis C. The side effects of BRM therapy often include flu-like symptoms such as chills, fever, muscle aches, weakness, loss of appetite, nausea, vomiting, and diarrhea. Some patients develop a rash, and some bleed or bruise easily. Interleukin therapy can cause swelling. Depending on the severity of these problems, patients may need to stay in the hospital during treatment. These side effects are usually short-term and go gradually away after treatment stops.

Biopsy: To take a small sample of tissue for analysis.

Cervix: The cervix is the lower, narrow part of the uterus (womb). The uterus, a hollow, pear-shaped organ, is located in a woman's lower abdomen, between the bladder and the rectum. The cervix forms a canal that opens into the vagina, which leads to the outside of the body.

Coccyx: A small curved bone emerging from the sacrum at the bottom of the backbone. This bone, also known as the tailbone, is the posterior connection of the pubococcygeal muscle.

Colposcopy: A procedure using a binocular microscope (colposcope) for detailed inspection of the vulvar, vagina, and cervix under magnification.

Condyloma: Flat or wart-like growths around the anus, vulva, or glans penis caused by the human papilloma virus (HPV).

Connective tissue: As the name implies, this tissue connects various structures of the body together. Connective tissue is found in great abundance within the skin and muscles. It is primarily composed of protein, collagen, and cells called fibroblasts.

Cystitis: This is a general term for inflammation of the bladder

Cystoscope: An instrument used to look inside the bladder. Both rigid and flexible cystoscopes are available. The majority of urological procedures are performed through rigid cystoscopy. A flexible cystoscope usually has a smaller diameter, and its tip bends in different directions to allow visualization of the bladder wall. This type of cystoscope is usually used for diagnostic purposes.

Cytokines: Small proteins released by cells that have a specific effect on the interactions between cells, on communications between cells, or on the behavior of cells. The cytokines include the interleukins, lymphokines, and cell signal molecules, such as the tumor necrosis factor and the interferons, which trigger inflammation and respond to infections.

Discs: Shorthand for intervertebral discs, the disk-shaped pieces of specialized tissue that separate the bones of the spinal column. The center of each disc, called the nucleus, is soft, springy, and receives the shock of standing, walking, running, etc. The outer ring of the disc, called the *annulus* (Latin for "ring"), provides structure and strength. The annulus consists of a complex series of interwoven layers of fibrous tissue that hold the nucleus in place. The nuclear tissue located in the center of the disc can be placed under so much pressure that it can cause the annulus to rupture. When the disc has herniated or ruptured, it may create pressure against one or more of the spinal nerves, which can cause pain, weakness, or numbness.

Dysesthesia: An altered state of unpleasant sensation.

Dysesthetic vulvodynia: A form of vulvodynia marked by chronic, diffuse, unprovoked burning, stinging, or rawness in the vulva.

Dyspareunia: This term refers to pain during intercourse. Pain occurring at the opening of the vagina, the introitus, during penetration, is referred to as introital dyspareunia, and pain inside the vagina during thrusting is referred to as deep dyspareunia.

Dysuria: Urethral pain (usually burning) during urination.

Endometriosis: A condition where endometrium (the lining of the uterus) is found in other parts of the body. This tissue has the ability to bleed just as uterine tissue does during the menstrual cycle. Symptoms of endometriosis vary depending upon the location of the "implants."

Endoscopy: The examination of internal bodily structures with the aid of special instruments called endoscopes. Cytoscopy and laparoscopy are forms of endoscopy.

Epidemiology: The study of the source(s), prevalence, and distribution of disease within a given population.

Erythema: A redness of the skin resulting from inflammation—for example, sunburn.

Estrogen: The hormone responsible for many female sex characteristics such as breast development, the menstrual cycle, and maintenance of the vaginal lining. This hormone is also produced in men and in some plants.

Fibromyalgia: A syndrome defined by specific points of tenderness along the muscles and joints of the body and by sleep disorder.

Hashimoto's thyroiditis: Inflammation of the thyroid gland. The inflamed thyroid gland can release an excess of thyroid hormones into the bloodstream, resulting in a temporary hyperthyroid state. Once the thyroid gland is depleted of thyroid hormones, the patient commonly goes through a hypothyroid (low thyroid) phase. This phase can last three to six months until the thyroid gland fully recovers.

Herpes simplex virus (HSV): A family of viruses. The term *herpes* also refers to infection with one of the human herpes viruses, especially herpes simplex types 1 and 2. Herpes simplex type 1 (HSV-1) typically causes cold sores and fever blisters in the mouth and around it. Herpes simplex type 2 (HSV-2) typically causes genital herpes, a sexually transmitted disease (STD). Genital herpes is characterized by sores in the genital area. Both herpes simplex types 1 and 2 may cause lesions in the oral, genital, or other areas. They can cause systemic disease including encephalitis (infection of the brain) in someone who is immunodeficient. The treatment of infection with herpes simplex infections is by antiviral medication.

Histamine: A chemical released from mast cells (specialized inflammatory cells) that stimulates inflammation.

Histology: Microscopic study of the body's tissues.

Human papilloma virus (HPV): A family of over sixty viruses responsible for causing warts. The majority of human papilloma viruses produce warts on the hands, fingers, and even the face. Most of these viruses are innocuous, nothing more than cosmetic concerns. Several types of HPV, however, are confined primarily to the moist skin of the genitals, producing genital warts, and some subtypes elevate the risk for cancer of the cervix, vagina, and vulva. These latter viruses are sexually transmitted.

Hyperesthesia: Heightened sensitivity to a given stimulus in vulvar pain disorder. The vulva is thought to be hyperesthetic; thus the feeling of discomfort in the vulva occurs with only small amounts irritation.

Hypoxia: A lack of oxygen delivered to tissues, which may result in discomfort, tissue death, or abnormal functioning.

Incontinence: The unwanted leakage of urine or fecal matter.

Inflammation: A physiological response to infection, irritation, or injury. The cardinal signs are redness (rubor), heat (calor), swelling (tumor), and pain (dolor). This process is the result of proteins, called cytokines, causing changes in blood flow, blood vessel fluid exchange, and activation of white blood cells. The specifics of the reaction depend on the precipitating cause. The condition may resolve or develop to become "chronic."

Interferon: *See* Biological response modifiers.

Interleukin: *See* Biological response modifiers.

Interstitial cystitis: Disease of oversensitivity of the urinary bladder, marked by inflammation and ulceration, causing urinary urgency, frequency and suprapubic pain.

Introitus: The opening of the vagina.

Irritable bowel syndrome (IBS): A common gastrointestinal disorder (also called spastic colitis, mucus colitis, or nervous colon syndrome), IBS is an abnormal condition of gut contractions (motility) characterized by abdominal pain, bloating, mucus in stools, and irregular bowel habits with alternating diarrhea and constipation—symptoms that tend to be chronic and wax and wane over the years. Although IBS can cause chronic recurrent discomfort, it does not lead to any serious organ problems. Diagnosis usually involves excluding other illnesses. Treatment is directed toward relief of symptoms (and includes a high fiber diet and avoidance of caffeine and milk products).

Laparoscopy: A surgical procedure in which a special viewing intrument called a laparoscope is inserted into the abdominal cavity through a small incision. In this way the abdominal cavity can be examined, and if necessary, laparoscopic surgery can be performed by inserting specially designed instruments through other small incisions.

Lichen: A broad category encompassing all dermatological disorders resulting in lichenification, a term which comes from the fact that these conditions have the appearance of lichens (a mixture of algae and fungi) in nature.

Lichenification: Thick, leathery skin, sometimes the result of scratching and rubbing. With prolonged rubbing or scratching, the outer layer of the skin (the epidermis) becomes thicker, and this results in exaggeration of the normal skin markings, giving the skin a leathery, bark-like appearance. Lichenification is a common consequence of atopic dermatitis (eczema) and other pruritic (itchy) disorders. It may also arise on seemingly normal skin.

Lichen planus: A common condition that causes itchy pink/purple flat spots on the skin, usually on the wrists, shins, and back. When it occurs in the mouth or on the genitals, it appears as thin red patches with (sometimes) thin white "lacy" borders. It can cause an extremely inflammatory vaginal change, which may result in scarring. Treatment is with topical steroids.

Lupus: A chronic inflammatory condition caused by an autoimmune disease. Patients with lupus have unusual antibodies in their blood that are targeted against their own body tissues. Lupus can cause disease of the skin, heart, lungs, kidneys, joints, and nervous system. When only the skin is involved, the condition is called discoid lupus. When internal organs are involved, the condition is called systemic lupus erythematosus (SLE). Up to 10 percent of persons with discoid lupus eventually develop the systemic form of lupus (SLE). SLE is eight times more common in women than men. The causes of SLE are unknown. However, heredity, viruses, ultraviolet light, and drugs may all play a role.

Mast cells: Inflammatory cells that contain "packets" of chemicals that stimulate inflammation such as prostaglandins, histamine, and leukotrienes.

Mucosa: The thin lining of many body surfaces that secretes a protective, slimy substance called *mucin*.

Neuralgia: Pain along the course of a nerve.

Neuroma: A benign tumor that arises in nerve cells.

Neuropathic pain: Pain caused by damage to nerve cells.

Neurostimulation or neuromodulation: A technique where nerves are electrically stimulated. This procedure has been found to be useful in the management of many pain syndromes. Neuromodulation also has recently been used urologically to treat bladders that function abnormally.

Nociceptive pain: Pain arising from continuing inflammatory tissue damage.

Opioids: This is a class of medication derived from opiates and used to manage chronic pain disorders. Because of the addictive potential of these drugs and other serious side effects, doctors tend to limit their use.

Oxalate: A chemical substance commonly found in foods of plant origin. Oxalates in the urine (hyperoxaluria) may be a contributory factor to vulvodynia. They can also cause kidney stones.

Pelvic floor: A "hammock" of muscle and connective tissue that sits at the base of the pelvis and supports the pelvic organs. The pelvic floor has numerous functions related to defecation, urination, and sexual intercourse.

Pelvic floor dysfunction: Abnormal function (spasm) or weakness of the muscles comprising the pelvic floor. This is frequently associated with complaints of lower back pain, constipation, poor urinary flow, pain with sexual intercourse, or generalized pelvic pain.

Perineum: The region between the vagina and anus or the scrotum and anus.

pH: A measurement of the acidity or alkalinity of a solution. The lower the pH, the more acidic the solution. The higher the pH, the more alkaline the solution. A pH of 7 is neither alkaline nor acidic (it is neutral).

Placebo: Also known as a "sugar pill," any physiologically inactive substance that is not effective for treating any disease process but can appear to help because the patient believes it is effective. This favorable response is called the "placebo effect."

Postvoid residual (PVR): The amount of urine that remains in the bladder after urination.

Prostatodynia (male chronic pelvic pain syndrome, category IIIB): The literal translation is "prostate pain"; in this instance, the pain, which mimics prostatitis, is actually caused by spasm of the pelvic floor muscles.

Pubis: The bone making up the lower and front section of the pelvic bones. It is the bone that lies directly above the vaginal opening. The fatty layer covering this bone is known as the mons pubis.

Pubococcyegus: This is one of the muscles of the pelvic floor which extends from the bottom of the pubic bone back to the coccyx bone and forms a sling, or a hammock, of muscle which surrounds the urethra, vagina, and anus.

Recurrent urinary tract infection: Urinary tract infections that occur more than two to three times per year.

Reflex sympathetic dystrophy (RSD): A condition characterized by diffuse pain, swelling, and limitation of movement following an injury, such as a fracture in an arm or leg, in which the symptoms are way out of proportion to the injury and may linger long after the injury has healed.

Sarcoidosis: A disease of unknown origin that causes small lumps (granulomas) due to chronic inflammation to develop in a great range of body tissues. Sarcoidosis can appear in almost any body organ including the vulva. In the majority of cases, the granulomas clear up with or without treatment. In cases where the granulomas do not heal and disappear, the tissues tend to remain inflamed and become scarred (fibrotic).

Sjogren's syndrome: An autoimmune disease that classically combines dry eyes, dry mouth, and another disease of the connective tissues, such as rheumatoid arthritis (most common), lupus, scleroderma, or polymyositis. About 90 percent of Sjogren's syndrome patients are female, usually in middle age or older. Sjogren's syndrome is an inflammatory disease of the glands and other tissues of the body. Inflammation of the lacrimal glands, which produce tears leads to decreased tears and dry eyes. Inflammation of the salivary glands, which produce saliva in the mouth, leads to dry mouth.

Sjogren's syndrome can consequently be complicated by infections of the eyes, breathing passages, and mouth. Sjogren's syndrome is typically associated with autoantibodies produced by the body, which are directed against a variety of body tissues.

Spermicide: Medications that kill sperm on contact. Usually used in conjunction with a condom or diaphragm for birth control.

Squamous cell carcinoma: Cancer that begins in squamous cells—thin, flat cells that look under the microscope like fish scales. Squamous cells are found in the tissue that forms the surface of the skin, mucous membranes, and the lining of the hollow organs of the body, and the passages of the respiratory and digestive tracts. Squamous cell carcinomas may arise in any of these tissues.

Substance P: A small molecule found in certain nerve fibers. Substance P appears to stimulate inflammation and also functions in the transmission of pain within the nervous system.

Suprapubic: Above the pubic bone.

TENS (transcutaneous electrical nerve stimulation): A method of pain management using a low level of electrical stimulation applied to the body's surface.

Tricyclic antidepressants (TCA): One of a class of medications used to treat depression. The tricyclic antidepressants are also used for some forms of anxiety, fibromyalgia, and the control of chronic pain. "Tricyclic" refers to the presence of three rings in the chemical structure of these drugs. Amitriptyline (Elavil) and nortriptyline (Pamelor) are most commonly used in the treatment of vulvodynia.

Trigone: The base of the bladder. *Trigonitis* is a nonspecific term denoting redness (possibly inflammation) in this region.

Uncomplicated urinary tract infection: A urinary tract infection that is usually superficial, easily treated, and not associated with structural or functional abnormalities of the urinary tract.

Urethra: The tube that allows urine to exit the bladder. The opening where the urine comes out is called the *urethral meatus*.

Urethral dilation: A "stretching" of the urethra performed by inserting an instrument called a urethral dilator. In many instances, progressively larger urethral dilators are inserted into the urethra until the desired degree of dilation is achieved.

Urethral meatus: The opening of the urethra; located at the end of the penis in males and just above the vaginal opening in females.

Urethral stenosis: A narrowing of the urethra.

Urethral syndrome: A poorly understood condition marked by urinary urgency and frequency and urethral pain. Most patients also complain of urethral burning or burning while urinating. Urethral syndrome is believed by many to be a form of interstitial cystitis.

Urethritis: Inflammation of the urethra.

Urinalysis: A basic characterization of the urine including such parameters as pH, urine concentration, the presence or absence of blood, white blood cells, and sugar. Many urinalyses also include a microscopic review (called a *microscopic urinalysis*).

Vagina: The muscular canal extending from the introitus to the cervix.

Vaginismus: Painful spasm of the vagina causing severe pain with sexual intercourse.

Vaginitis: Inflammation of the vagina. Vaginitis may be caused by fungus (yeast), bacteria, hormonal imbalance, chemical irritation/allergy, or conditions such as lichen planus. A woman with this condition may have itching or burning and may notice a discharge. Vaginitis is a common condition.

Vestibule (of the vulva): The vestibule contains the urethral opening (meatus), the opening of the vagina (the introitus), Skene's glands, Bartholin's glands, and minor vestibular glands. This area extends from the clitoris to the bottom of the vaginal opening and laterally to the inner aspect of the labia minora.

Vestibulectomy: Excision of the vulvar vestibule.

Vestibulitis: A form of vulvodynia marked by point tenderness limited to the vulvar vestibule and occurring only with pressure, resulting in pain at the vaginal opening with touch or attempted penetration. This condition is also known as vulvar vestibulitis syndrome.

Vestibulodynia: A condition in which vulvar pain is localized to the vulvar vestibule and occurs only on touch or pressure, causing introital dyspareunia.

Void: To urinate.

Vulva: The external female genital region (see figure 3 in chapter 2) including the mons pubis, labia majora and minora, the vaginal vestibule, and the clitoris.

Vulvar intraepithelial neoplasa (VIN): A precancerous abnormality of the cells and architecture of the skin of the vulva. Probably caused by human papilloma virus (HPV). Highly curable (noninvasive). Also known as squamous intraepithelial neoplasia (SIL), usually divided into "low-grade" SIL (mild changes) and "high-grade" SIL (moderate to severe changes, including carcinoma in situ).

Vulvectomy: Excision of the vulva followed by surgical reconstruction of the region.

Vulvodynia: A general term literally meaning "vulvar pain." Vulvar pain can develop from many medical conditions, including vaginal infections, estrogen loss, and dermatological problems. In some instances, there is no apparent cause.

Yeast infection: Yeast infections occur most frequently in moist areas of the body. Overgrowth of yeast can affect the skin (yeast rash), mouth (thrush), digestive tract, esophagus, vagina (vaginitis), and other areas. Various species of yeast may cause infections. Generally, the most common is Candida albicans. Various nonalbicans Candida species (C. glabrata, C. tropicalis, C. krusei) and other fungi, such as Trichosporon, may also cause infection.

Appendix B

Resources

Vulvar Pain Treatment Centers

Gae Rodke, M.D., F.A.C.O.G.
146 Central Park West
Suite 1G
New York, NY 10023
(212) 496-9800

Center for Vulvovaginal Disorders
3 Washington Circle, NW, Suite 100
Washington, DC 20037
(202) 728-2997

Stewart-Forbes Vulvovaginal Center
291 Independence Drive
West Roxbury, MA 02467
(617) 541-6671

Vulvovaginal Organizations

National Vulvodynia Association
P.O. Box 4491
Silver Spring, MD 20914-4491
(301) 299-0775
www.nva.org

U.S. Vulvar Health Awareness Initiative
P.O. Box 6762
Bloomington, IN 47407
http://www.vulvarhealth.org/

Vulval Pain Society
P.O. Box 514
Slough
Berks SL1 2BP
UK
http://www.vul-pain.dircon.co.uk

Professional Organizations

American Academy of Pain Management
13947 Mono Way, no. A
Sonora, CA 95370
(209) 533-9744
www.aapainmanage.org

American Academy of Pain Medicine
4700 W. Lake Avenue
Glenview, IL 60025
(847) 375-4731
www.painmed.org

American Board of Dermatology
1 Ford Plaza
Detroit, MI 48202-3450
(313) 874-1088
www.abderm.org

American Board of Internal Medicine
510 Walnut Street, Suite 1700
Philadelphia, PA 19106-2246
(800) 441-2246
www.abim.org

American Board of Pathology
P.O. Box 25915
Tampa, FL 33622-5915
(813) 286-2444
www.abpath.org

American College of Nurse Practitioners
1111 19th Street, NW, Suite 404
Washington, DC 20036
(202) 659-2190
www.nurse.org/acnp

American College of Obstetricians and Gynecologists
409 12th Street, SW
P.O. Box 96920
Washington, DC 20090-6920
www.acog.org

American Physical Therapy Association
1111 N. Fairfax Street
Alexandria, VA 22314-1488
(800) 999-2782
www.apta.org

American Society for Colposcopy and Cervical Pathology
20 W. Washington Street, Suite 1
Hagerstown, MD 21740
(800) 787-7227
www.asccp.org

American Urological Association
1120 N. Charles Street
Baltimore, MD 21201
(410) 727-1100
www.auanet.org

Association for Applied Psychophysiology and Biofeedback
10200 West 44th Avenue, Suite 304
Wheat Ridge, CO 80033-2840
(303) 422-8436
http://AAPB.org

International and American Association of Clinical Nutritionists
16775 Addison Road, suite 100
Addison, TX 75001
(972) 407-9089
www.iaacn.org

International Society for the Study of Vulvovaginal Disease
8814 Peppergrass Lane
Waxhaw, NC 28173
(704) 814-9493
www.issvd.org

Government Information

Centers for Disease Control and Prevention
1600 Clifton Road
Atlanta, GA 30333
(404) 639-3311
www.cdc.gov

National Institute of Child Health and Human Development
Building 31, Room 2A32, MSC 2425
31 Center Drive
Bethesda, MD 20892-2425
www.nichd.nih.gov

**National Institute of Child Health and Human Development
Clearinghouse (Institute Funding Vulvodynia Research)**
P.O. Box 3006
Rockville, MD 20847
(800) 370-2943
nichdclearinghouse@mail.nih.gov

**National Institute of Diabetes and Digestive and Kidney Diseases
(NIDDK)**
Office of Communications and Public Liason, NIDDK, NIH
31 Center Drive, MSC 2560
Bethesda, MD 20892-2560
www.niddk.nih.gov

National Institutes of Health
Office of Research on Women's Health
Building 1, Room 201
9000 Rockville Pike
Bethesda, MD 20892-0161
(301) 402-1770
www4.od.nih.gov/orwh/
www.clinicaltrials.gov

The National Institutes of Health, through its National Library of Medicine, has developed www.clinicaltrials.gov to provide patients, family members, and members of the public with current information about clinical research studies.

U.S. Food and Drug Administration
5600 Fisher Lane
Rockville, MD 20857-0001
(888) 463-6332
www.fda.gov

Organizations for Vulvodynia-Related Conditions

Urology-Related Information

American Foundation for Urologic Disease/The Bladder Health Council
1128 N. Charles Street
Baltimore, MD 21201
(800) 242-2383
www.afud.org

Interstitial Cystitis Association
51 Monroe Street, Suite 1402
Rockville, MD 20850
(800) HELP-ICA
www.IChelp.org

Interstitial Cystitis Network
4773 Sonoma Highway, PMB no. 125
Santa Rosa, CA 95409
(707) 538-9442
www.ic-network.org

National Association for Continence
P.O. Box 8306
Spartanburg, SC 29305-8306
(846) 579-7900

National Bladder Foundation
P.O. Box 1095
Ridgefield, CT 06877
(203) 431-0005
www.bladder.org

Prostatitis Foundation
1063 30th Street, Box 8
Smithshire, IL 614478
(888) 891-4200
www.prostatitis.org

The Simon Foundation for Continence
P.O. Box 85-F
Wilmette, IL 60091
(800) 23-SIMON
www.simonfoundation.org

Respiratory-Related Information

Allergy and Asthma Network/Mothers of Asthmatics, Inc.
2751 Prosperity Avenue, Suite 150
Fairfax, VA 22030-2709
(800) 878-4403
www.aanma.org

Asthma & Allergy Foundation of America
1125 15th Street, NW, Suite 502
Washington, DC 20005
(800) 727-8462
www.aafa.org

Gastrointestinal-Related Information

Crohn's and Colitis Foundation of America, Inc.
National Headquarters
444 Park Avenue South, 11th Floor
New York, NY 10016
(800) 932-2423
www.ccfa.org

International Foundation for Functional Gastrointestinal Disorders (IFFGD)
P.O. Box 17864
Milwaukee, WI 53217
(888) 964-2001
www.iffgd.org

Irritable Bowel Syndrome Association
1440 Whalley Avenue, no. 145
New Haven, CT 06515
(416) 932-3311
www.ibsassociation.org

Gynecological-Related Information

Endometriosis Association, Inc.
8585 N. 76th Place
Milwaukee, WI 53223
(800) 992-3636
www.endometriosisassn.org

North American Menopause Society
5900 Landerbrook Road, Suite 195
Mayfield Heights, OH 44124
(440) 442-7550
www.menopause.org

Autoimmune-Related Information

American Autoimmune Related Diseases Association, Inc.
22100 Gratiot Avenue
East Detroit, MI 48021
(810) 776-3900
www.aarda.org

American Fibromyalgia Syndrome Association, Inc.
6389 E. Tanque Verde Road, Suite D
Tucson, AZ 85715
(520) 773-1570
www.afsafund.org

Arthritis Foundation
1330 W. Peachtree
Atlanta, GA 30309
(800) 283-7800
www.arthritis.org

The CFIDS Association of America, Inc.
P.O. Box 220398
Charlotte, NC 28222-0398
(800) 44-CFIDS
www.cfids.org

Fibromyalgia Association of Greater Washington
13203 Valley Drive
Woodbridge, VA 22191-1531
(703) 551-4160
www.fmagw.org

The Fibromyalgia Network
P.O. Box 31750
Tucson, AZ 85751-1750
(800) 853-2929
www.fmnetnews.com

Fibromyalgia Wellness Newsletter (Arthritis Foundation)
P.O. Box 921907
Norcross, GA 30010-1907
(877) 775-0343

International Fibromyalgia Exchange
Deutsche Fibromyalgie-Vereinigung Postfach 1308
71536 Murrhardt, Germany
www.Weiss.de/Fibro.htm

Lupus Foundation of America
4 Research Place, Suite 180
Rockville, MD 20850-3226
(800) 558-0121
www.lupus.org

Massachusetts CFIDS Association
P.O. Box 690305
Quincy, MA 02269-0305
(617) 471-5559
www.masscfids.org

The Mastocytosis Society, Inc.
4771 Waynes Trace Road
Hamilton, OH 45011
(513) 726-4642
www.mastocytosis.com

National Sjogren's Syndrome Association
5815 N. Black Canyon Highway, Suite 103
Phoenix, AZ 85015-2200
(800) 395-NSSA

Sjogren's Syndrome Foundation
333 N. Broadway
Jericho, NY 11753
(516) 933-6365
www.sjogrens.com

Dermatology-Related Information

National Lichen Sclerosus Support Group (UK)
2 Ivy House
Wantage Road
Great Shefford
Berkshire RG17 7DA
UK
www.lichensclerosus.org

Endocrinology-Related Information

Thyroid Foundation of America
350 Ruth Sleeper Hall, RSL 350
40 Parkman Street
Boston, MA 02114-2698
(800) 832-8321
www.tsh.org

Headache-Related Disorders

American Council for Headache Education (ACHE)
19 Mantua Road
Mt. Royal, NJ 08061
(800) 255-2243
www.achenet.org

The National Headache Foundation
(888) NHF-5552
www.headaches.org

Sex Therapy and Information Organizations

American Association of Sexuality Educators, Counselors and Therapists
P.O. Box 5488
Richmond, VA 23220-0488
www.aasect.org

American Board of Sexology
American Academy of Clinical Sexologists
2180 Park Avenue North, Suite 300
Winter Park, FL 32789
(407) 645-1641
www.sexologist.org
www.sexhelp.org

Sexuality Information and Education Council of the U.S.
130 W. 42nd Street, Suite 350
New York, NY 10036-7802
(212) 819-9770
www.siecus.org

Society for the Scientific Study of Sexuality
P.O. Box 416
Allentown, PA 18105-0416
(610) 530-2483
www.sexscience.org

World Association of Sexology
1300 S. Second Street, Suite 180
Minneapolis, MN 55414
(612) 625-1500
www.tc.umn.edu/~colem001/was/

Psychotherapy/Counseling Organizations

American Association for Marriage and Family Therapy
1133 15th Street, NW, Suite 300
Washington, DC 20005-2710
(202) 452-0109
www.aamft.org

American Psychiatric Association
1400 K Street, NW
Washington, DC 20005
(888) 357-7924
www.psych.org

American Psychiatric Nurses Association
Colonial Place Three
2107 Wilson Boulevard, Suite 300-A
Arlington, VA 22201-3042
www.apna.org

American Psychological Association
750 First Street, NE
Washington, DC 20002-4242
(800) 374-2721
www.apa.org

National Association of Social Workers
750 First Street, NE, Suite 700
Washington, DC 20002-4241
(800) 638-8799
www.naswdc.org

Pain Organizations

American Chronic Pain Association
P.O. Box 850
Rocklin, CA 95677
(916) 632-0922
www.theacpa.org

American Pain Foundation
201 N. Charles, Suite 710
Baltimore, MD 21201-4111
www.painfoundation.org

American Pain Society /International Association for the Study of Pain
4700 W. Lake Avenue
Glenview, IL 60025
(847) 375-4715
www.ampainsoc.org

International Pelvic Pain Society
Women's Medical Plaza, Suite 402
2006 Brookwood Medical Center Drive
Birmingham, AL 35209
(800) 624-9676
www.pelvicpain.org

National Chronic Pain Outreach Association
P.O. Box 274
Millboro, VA 24460-9606
(540) 862-9437
www.paincare.org

National Foundation for the Treatment of Pain
1330 Skyline Drive, no. 21
Monterey, CA 93940
(831) 655-8812
www.paincare.org

Other Helpful Organizations

National Organization of Rare Diseases
P.O. Box 8923
New Fairfield, CT 06812-8923
(800) 999-6673
www.rarediseases.org

Reflex Sympathetic Dystrophy Syndrome Association of America
116 Haddon Avenue, Suite D
Haddonfield, NJ 08033
(609) 795-8845

TMJ Association (Temporal-Mandibular Joint Diseases)
P.O. Box 26770
Milwaukee, WI 54226
(414) 259-3223
www.tmj.org

United Ostomy Association
19772 MacArthur Boulevard, Suite 200
Irvine, CA 92612
(800) 826-0826
www.uoa.org

Well Spouse Foundation
P.O. Box 30093
Elkins Park, PA 19027
(631) 661-0421
www.wellspouse.org

Special Concerns of Women

Centers for Disease Control and Prevention
(800) 311-3435
www.cdc.gov

Center for Patient Advocacy
(800) 846-7444
www.patientadvocacy.org

Food and Drug Administration
(888) 463-6332
www.fda.gov

HERS Foundation—Hysterectomy Educational Resources and Services
422 Bryn Mawr Avenue
Bala Cynwyd, PA 19004
(610) 667-7757
www.nafc.org

National Center for Complementary and Alternative Medicine
(888) 644-6226
altmed.od.nih.gov/nccam

National Library of Medicine
(888) 346-3656
www.nlm.nih.gov

Society for the Advancement of Women's Health Research
1828 L Street, NW, Suite 625
Washington, DC 20036
(202) 223-8224
www.womens-health.org

Women's International Pharmacy
13925 W. Meeker Boulevard, Suite 13
Sun City West, AZ 85375
(800) 279-5708
www.womensinternational.com

World Foundation for Medical Studies in Female Health
405 Main Street
Port Washington, NY 11050
(516) 944-7340
www.wffh.org

Disability/Social Security Information

Americans with Disabilities Act Information
(800) 514-0301

**National Organization of Social Security Claimants'
Representatives**
6 Prospect Street
Midland Park, NJ 07432
(800) 431-2804

Social Security Administration
Write or call your local office (look in your telephone book under
U.S. Government, Department of Health and Human Services) or call
(800) 234-5772 or visit the Web site at www.ssa.gov

References

Ashman, R.B., and A.K. Ott. 1989. Autoimmunity as a factor in recurrent vaginal candidosis and the minor vestibular gland syndrome. *Journal of Reproductive Medicine* 34:264-66.

Baggish, M.S., E.H.M. Sze, and R. Johnson. 1997. Urinary oxalate excretion and its role in vulvar pain syndrome. *American Journal of Obstetrics and Gynecology* 177:507-11.

Bazin, S., et al. 1994. Vulvar vestibulitis syndrome: An exploratory case-control study. *American Journal of Obstetrics and Gynecology* 83:47-50.

Bergeron, S., et al. 1994. Vulvar vestibulitis: Lack of evidence for a human papillomavirus etiology. *Journal of Reproductive Medicine* 39:936-38.

Bergeron, S., et al. 2001. A randomized comparison of group cognitive-behavioral therapy, surface electromyographic biofeedback, and vestibulectomy in the treatment of dyspareunia resulting from vulvar vestibulitis. *Pain* 91:297-306.

Binik, I., and S. Bergeron. 2001. *NVA News* 6(3):1–7.

Bohm-Starke, N. 2001. Psychophysiologic evidence for nociceptor sensitization in vulvar vestibulitis syndrome. Presented at the sixteenth world congress meeting of the International Society for the Study of Vulvovaginal Disease, 30 September–4 October, in Sintra, Portugal.

Bohm-Starke, N., et al. 1998. Increased intraepithelial innervation in women with vulvar vestibulitis syndrome. *Gynecologic and Obstetric Investigation* 46:256-60.

Bornstein, J. 2001. A mathematical model for the histopathologic diagnosis of vulvar vestibulitis, based on a histomorphometric study of innervation and mast cell activation. Presented at the sixteenth world congress meeting of the International Society for the Study of Vulvovaginal Disease, 30 September–4 October, in Sintra, Portugal.

Bornstein, J., B. Pascal, and H. Abramovici. 1993. Intramuscular beta-interferon treatment for severe vulvar vestibulitis. *Journal of Reproductive Medicine* 38:117-20.

Bornstein, J., et al. 1995. Perineoplasty compared with vestibuloplasty for severe vulvar vestibulitis. *British Journal of Obstetrics and Gynaecology* 102:652-55.

Bornstein, J., et al. 1997. Predicting the outcome of surgical treatment of vulvar vestibulitis. *American Journal of Obstetrics and Gynecology* 89:695-98.

Catalano, E.M., and K.N. Hardin. 1996. *The Chronic Pain Control Workbook*. Oakland, Calif.: New Harbinger Publications.

Chaim, W., et al. 1996. Vulvar vestibulitis subjects undergoing surgical intervention: A descriptive analysis and histopathological correlates. *European Journal of Obstetrics and Gynecology and Reproductive Biology* 68:165-68.

Davis, M., E.R. Eshelman, and M. McKay. 2000. *The Relaxation and Stress Reduction Workbook*. Oakland, Calif.: New Harbinger Publications.

Denbow, M.L., and M.A. Byrne. 1998. Prevalence, causes and outcome of vulvar pain in a genitourinary medicine clinic population. *International Journal of STD and AIDS* 9:88-91.

Dennerstein, G.J., et al. 1994. Human papillomavirus vulvitis: A new disease or an unfortunate mistake? *British Journal of Obstetrics and Gynecology* 101:992.

Dodson, Betty. 1996. *Sex for One: The Joy of Self-Loving*. New York: Crown Publishing.

Edwards, A., and F. Wiojnarowska. 1998. The vulval pain syndromes. *International Journal STD AIDS* 9:74.

Foster, D.C. 2001. Fibroblast heterogeneity leads to differential production of cycle-oxygenate 1, 2 and prostaglandin E2 in vulvar vestibulitis (vulvodynia). Presented at the sixteenth world congress meeting of the International Society for the Study of Vulvovaginal Disease, 30 September–4 October, in Sintra, Portugal.

Foster, D.C., and J.D. Hasday. 1997. Elevated tissue levels of interleukin-1 beta and tumor necrosis factor-alpha in vulvar vestibulitis. *Obstetrics and Gynecology* 89:291-96.

Foster, D.C., and K. Duguid. 1998. Open label study of oral desipramine and topical lidocaine for the treatment of vulvar vestibulitis. Abstract delivered at conference on mechanism and treatment of neuropathic pain, 15–20 April, in Rochester, New York.

Foster, D.C., et al. 1995. Long-term outcome of perineoplasty for vulvar vestibulitis. *Journal of Women's Health* 4:669-75.

Friedrich, E.G., Jr. 1987. Vulvar vestibulitis syndrome. *Journal of Reproductive Medicine* 32:110-14.

Gatchel, R.J., et al. 1995. The dominant role of psychological risk factors in the development of chronic low back pain disability. *Spine* 20:2702-2709.

Glazer, H.I. 2000. Dysesthetic vulvodynia: Long-term follow-up after treatment with surface electromyography-assisted pelvic floor muscle rehabilitation. *Journal of Reproductive Medicine* 45:798-802.

Glazer, H.I., et al. 1998. Electromyographic comparisons of the pelvic floor in women with dysesthetic vulvodynia and asymptomatic women. *Journal of Reproductive Medicine* 43:959-62.

Glazer, H.I., G. Rodke, et al. 1995. Treatment of vulvar vestibulitis syndrome with electromyographic biofeedback of pelvic floor musculature. *Journal of Reproductive Medicine* 40:283-90.

Goetsch, M.F. 1991. Vulvar vestibulitis: prevalence and historic features in a general gynecologic practice population. *American Journal of Obstetrics and Gynecology* 164:1609-16.

————. 1996. Simplified surgical revision of the vulvar vestibule for vulvar vestibulitis. *American Journal of Obstetrics and Gynecology* 174:1701-7.

————. 1999. Postpartum dyspareunia: An unexplored problem. *Journal of Reproductive Medicine* 44:963-68.

Haefner, H., and R. Kaufman. 1998. A classical approach to vulvar disease. CD-ROM. Washington, D.C.: American College of Obstetricians and Gynecologists.

Hitchcock, L.D., B.R. Ferrell, and M. McCaffrey. 1994. The experience of chronic nonmalignant pain. *Journal of Pain Symptom Management* 1994 Jul:9(5):312-18

Kegel, A. 1948. Progressive exercise in the functional restoration of the perineal muscles. *American Journal of Obstetrics and Gynecology* 56:238-48.

Kelly, H.A. 1928. Dyspareunia. In *Gynecology*, edited by H.A. Kelly. New York: D. Appleton and Company.

Klein, M., and R. Robbins. 1998. *Let Me Count the Ways.* New York: Tarcher Putnam.

Laumann, E., et al. 1994. *The Social Organization of Sexuality.* Chicago: University of Chicago Press.

Ledger, W.J., et al. 1996. Vulvar vestibulitis: A complex clinical entity. *Infectious Diseases in Obstetrics and Gynecology* 4:269.

Ledger, W.J., J. Jeremias, and S.S. Witkin. 2000. Testing for high-risk human papillomavirus types will become a standard of clinical care. *American Journal of Obstetrics and Gynecology* 182 (4):860-65.

Mann, M.S., et al. 1992. Vulvar vestibulitis: Significant clinical variables and treatment outcome. *Obstetrics and Gynecology* 79:122-25.

Marinoff, S. 1995. Vulvodynia: A perplexing disorder. *NVA News* 1(1):1-9.

————. 1996. Vulvodynia and pregnancy. *NVA News* 2(2):8-9.

Marinoff, S.C., and M.L.C. Turner. 1991. Vulvar vestibulitis syndrome: An overview. *American Journal of Obstetrics and Gynecology* 165:1228-33.

Marinoff, S.C., and M.L.C. Turner. 1992. Vulvar vestibulitis syndrome. *Dermatologic Clinic* 10:435-44.

McKay, M. 1990. Vulvar dermatoses: Common problems in dermatological and gynecological practice. *British Journal of Clinical Practice* 71(suppl):5-10.

Meana, M., et al. 1998a. Biopsychosocial profile of women with dyspareunia. *American Journal of Obstetrics and Gynecology* 90:583-89.

———. 1998b. Affect and marital adjustment in women's rating of dyspareunic pain. *Canadian Journal of Psychiatry* 43:381-85.

———. 1999. Psychosocial correlates of pain attribution in women with dyspareunia. *Psychosomatics* 40(6):497-502.

Neill, S.M., and C.M. Ridley. 1999. Vulvodynia. In *The Vulva*, edited by S.M. Neill and C.M. Ridley. Oxford, UK: Blackwell Scientific.

Nyirjesy, P. 2000. Vulvar vestibulitis syndrome: A post infectious entity. *Current Infectious Disease Reports* 2:531-35.

Perry, J.D., and B. Whipple. 1980. Two devices for the physiological measurement of sexual activity. Presented at the eastern region conference of the Society for the Scientific Study of Sex.

Pollin, I. 1995. *Taking Charge: Overcoming the Challenges of Long Term Illness.* New York: Times Books.

Powell, J., and F. Wojnarowska. 1999. Acupuncture for vulvodynia. *Journal of the Royal Society of Medicine* 92:579-81.

Reid, R., et al. 1995. Flashlamp-excited dye laser therapy of idiopathic vulvodynia is safe and efficacious. *American Journal of Obstetrics and Gynecology* 172:1684-1701.

Rodke, G. 2000. Vulvar conditions: Pregnancy and childbirth. *NVA News* 6(1):1-3.

Sadownik, L.A. 2000. Clinical profile of vulvodynia patients. *Journal of Reproductive Medicine* 45(8):679-84.

Sand Peterson, C., and K. Weismann. Isoprenosine improves symptoms in young females with chronic vulvodynia. *Acta Derm Venereol* (Stockholm) 76:404.

Sanders, C. L. and P. Mate. 1998. NIH holds conference on gender and pain. *NVA News* 4(2):1-11.

Skene, A. 1889. *Treatise on the Diseases of Women.* New York: Appleton and Company.

Slone, S., et al. 1999. Localization of chromogranin, synaptophysin, serotonin, and CXCR2 in neuroendocrine cells of the minor vestibular glands: An immunohistochemical study. *International Journal of Gynecological Pathology* 18:360-65.

Sobel, J.D., et al. 1998. Vulvovaginal candidiasis: Epidemiologic, diagnostic, and therapeutic considerations. *American Journal of Obstetrics and Gynecology* 178(2):203-11.

Solomons, C.C., M.H. Melmed, and S.M. Heitler. 1991. Calcium citrate for vulvar vestibulitis: a case report. *Journal of Reproductive Medicine* 36:879-82.

St. Amand, R.P. 1999. *What Your Doctor May Not Tell You About Fibromyalgia.* New York: Warner Books.

Stewart, E. 2001a. Vulvodynia: Diagnosing and managing generalized dysesthesia. *OBG Management* June:48-57.

———. 2001b. Vestibulodynia: Tracing and treating vulvar pain. *OBG Management* July:28-40.

Thomason, J.L. 1999. Vulvodynia: An update on a cryptic condition. *The Female Patient* August(suppl):20-24.

Turner, M.L., and S.C. Marinoff. 1988. Association of human papillomavirus with vulvodynia and the vulvar vestibulitis syndrome. *Journal of Reproductive Medicine* 33(6):533-37.

Wallis, M. 1996. *Just Another Woman's Problem.* Self-published.

White, G., M. Jantos, and H. Glazer. 1997. Establishing the diagnosis of vulvar vestibulitis. *Journal of Reproductive Medicine* 42: 157-60.

Wilkinson, E.J., et al. 1993. Vulvar vestibulitis is rarely associated with human papillomavirus infection types 6, 11, 16, or 18. *International Journal of Gynecological Pathology* 12:344-49.

Witkin, S.S., et al. 2000. Individual immunity and susceptibility to female genital tract infection. *American Journal of Obstetrics and Gynecology* 183:252-56.

Witkin, S.S., S. Gerber, and W.J. Ledger. 2002. Influence of interleukin-1 receptor antagonist gene polymorphism on disease. *Clinical Infectious Diseases* 34(2):204-9.

Index

ually transmitted diseases
(STDs), 25, 26, 34-35
Sjogren's syndrome, 171-172
Skene, Alexander, 55
Skene's glands, 15
Social Security information, 190
socioeconomic status, 33
Solomons, Clive, 59-60, 86
spermicide, 172
spinal cord stimulation (SCS),
127
squamous cell carcinoma, 172
St. John's Wort, 90
steroid injection therapy, 126
Stewart, Elizabeth, 94, 104
stress: managing, 109, 130;
vulvodynia symptoms and, 49
substance P, 172
support groups, 99
support services, 99
suprapubic area, 172
surface electromyography
(sEMG), 20, 65, 67, 76
surgery: for chronic pain,
127-128; for vestibulitis, 23,
90-91
survey on vulvodynia, 31-45

T

tai chi, 130
Taking Charge (Pollin), 117
tampons, 46
Tegretol, 80
therapeutic massage, 129

therapy. *See* psychotherapy;
sexual therapyt
oilet paper, 106
topical anesthetics, 44
traditional Chinese medicine,
129-130
transcutaneous electrical nerve
stimulation (TENS), 127, 172
trazodone hydrochloride, 89
*Treatise on the Diseases of
Women* (Skene), 55
treatments, 78-91, 95;
acupuncture, 79; antibiotics,
79-80; anticonvulsants, 80-81;
antidepressants, 88-90;
anti-inflammatories, 81;
anti-virals, 82; anxiolytics,
82; biofeedback, 82-83; for
chronic pain, 125-131;
estrogen therapy, 83-84;
immune system modulators,
85; low oxalate diet, 86-87;
pharmaceutical, 125-127;
surgical, 90-91, 127-128;
survey results on, 42-45;
tricyclic antidepressants,
88-89; vestibulectomy, 90-91
trichloroacetic acid (TCA), 22
tricyclic antidepressants, 20,
88-89, 159, 172
trigger points, 58-59
trigone, 172
Trilafon, 89
Trileptal, 81
Turner, Maria, 58, 103

Howard I. Glazer, Ph.D., is a Clinical Psychologist in New York City with a professional practice specializing in the treatment of vulvovaginal pain syndromes. He is a Clinical Associate Professor of Psychology in Psychiatry and in Obstetrics and Gynecology at Cornell University Medical College/New York Presbyterian Hospital. He is a member of the International Societ for the Study of Vulvovaginal Disease (ISSVD), the Medical Board of the National Vulvodynia Association (NVA), and the Editorial Advisory Board of the chronic pelvic pain section for OBGYN.net. Glazer provides individual clinical services, training workshops, and in-office specialty training, and he is actively involved in several multidisciplinary and multinational research projects.

Gae M. Rodke, M.D., FACOG, is a Clinical Assistant Professor of Obstetrics and Gynecology at Columbia University College of Physicians and Surgeons, and a Clinical Associate Attending Physician at St. Luke's Roosevelt Hospital Center. She is a fellow of the American College of Obstetricians and Gynecologists and of the International Society for the Study of Vulvovaginal Diseases. Dr. Rodke has been involved in pioneering research to establish a working model for vulvovaginal pain and to develop effective treatments for these disorders. She has published research articles, conducted grand rounds at several hospitals, presented at professional society meetings, and lectured to medical students in this field for over ten years.

Some Other
New Harbinger Titles

Talk to Me, Item 3317 $12.95

Romantic Intelligence, Item 3309 $15.95

Transformational Divorce, Item 3414 $13.95

The Rape Recovery Handbook, Item 3376 $15.95

Eating Mindfully, Item 3503 $13.95

Sex Talk, Item 2868 $12.95

Everyday Adventures for the Soul, Item 2981 $11.95

A Woman's Addiction Workbook, Item 2973 $18.95

The Daughter-In-Law's Survival Guide, Item 2817 $12.95

PMDD, Item 2833 $13.95

The Vulvodynia Survival Guide, Item 2914 $15.95

Love Tune-Ups, Item 2744 $10.95

The Deepest Blue, Item 2531 $13.95

The 50 Best Ways to Simplify Your Life, Item 2558 $11.95

Brave New You, Item 2590 $13.95

Loving Your Teenage Daughter, Item 2620 $14.95

The Hidden Feelings of Motherhood, Item 2485 $14.95

The Woman's Book of Sleep, Item 2418 $14.95

Pregnancy Stories, Item 2361 $14.95

The Women's Guide to Total Self-Esteem, Item 2418 $13.95

Thinking Pregnant, Item 2302 $13.95

The Conscious Bride, Item 2132 $12.95

Juicy Tomatoes, Item 2175 $13.95

Facing 30, Item 1500 $12.95

Call **toll free, 1-800-748-6273,** or log on to our online bookstore at **www.newharbinger.com** to order. Have your Visa or Mastercard number ready. Or send a check for the titles you want to New Harbinger Publications, Inc., 5674 Shattuck Ave., Oakland, CA 94609. Include $4.50 for the first book and 75¢ for each additional book, to cover shipping and handling. (California residents please include appropriate sales tax.) Allow two to five weeks for delivery.

Prices subject to change without notice.

Si:
9/58
→ 8/ Andrea
costume measurements

1600 7x
1888
3992
700

900
0
550
392